THE BALANCED

BODY

COMPASS

A Step By Step Guide To Food And Wellness

The Balanced Balanced Body compass

Copyright © 2025 by **LINDA SMITH**

All rights reserved. No part of this publication may be reproduced, distributed, or transmitted in any form or by any means, including photocopying, recording, or other electronic or mechanical methods, without the prior written permission of the publisher, except in the case of brief quotations embodied in critical reviews and certain other noncommercial uses permitted by copyright law.

Table of contents

THE 1

BALANCED 1

BODY 1

COMPASS ....Error! Bookmark not defined.

What is the Autoimmune Protocol (AIP)? 5

Goals of the AIP...6

How Does the AIP Work?.....................................6

The main food groups eliminated on the AIP include: 7

Allowable nutrient-dense, anti-inflammatory whole foods 8

Healing the Gut...9

Reintroduction Protocol 10

Chapter 1 12

RECIPE 12

SECTIONS 12

Quick and Easy Anti-Inflammatory Breakfast Recipes..13

Overnight oats, smoothies, egg dishes, etc............20

Make-ahead breakfast meal prep ideas 26

vegetarian and vegan AIP (Autoimmune Protocol) friendly breakfast options: 34

plant-based main dish recipes that are AIP-compliant: 40

grain-free vegetarian recipe 55

Chicken , turkey, and beef recipes 62

Poultry, meat, and potato dishes 72

The Balanced Balanced Body compass

3

seafood entrees 82

Potato and sweet potato sides...............................89

Sauces, condiments, and dressings 96

dairy-free dressings and sauces...........................101

Nut-free condiments 107

Dips and spreads..113

Fruit-Based treats, beverages, and teas 119

Anti-Inflammatory Chia Seed Pudding recipe:......125

hydrating herbal tea blends: 130

Chapter 2 136

28-Day..136

Meal Plan 136

weekly meal plans and shopping lists for the 28-day meal plan: 137

Sample meal combinations using the recipes from the 28-day meal plan: 141

Tips for batch cooking and prep on the AIP diet:..143

Reference 145

The Balanced Balanced Body compass

What is the Autoimmune Protocol (AIP)?

The Autoimmune Protocol (AIP) is a specialized diet and lifestyle program designed to help reduce inflammation, heal the gut, and ultimately put autoimmune diseases into remission. It is based on the principles of functional medicine and the idea that what we eat can have a profound impact on our immune system and overall health.

The AIP takes the Paleo diet as a starting point and eliminates even more potential food irritants and gut-damaging compounds. It strictly avoids foods like grains, legumes, dairy, eggs, nuts, seeds, nightshades (tomatoes, peppers, etc.), alcohol, and certain spices that may trigger inflammation or leaky gut.

By removing these inflammatory foods for a period of time, usually 28-90 days, the AIP allows the body to rest, recover, and start healing. The focus is on nutrient-dense, anti-inflammatory foods like vegetables, fruits, quality proteins, healthy fats, and safe spices/herbs.

The Balanced Balanced Body compass

Goals of the AIP

- Regulate the immune system response

- Repair the gut lining to heal leaky gut

- Identify personal food intolerances

- Reduce systemic inflammation

How Does the AIP Work?

The Autoimmune Protocol is designed to remove inflammatory and gut-irritating foods to allow the body to focus its energy on healing rather than constantly fighting off triggers. This temporary elimination diet provides a metabolic "reset" of sorts. During the elimination phase, typically lasting 30-90 days depending on individual needs, the following food groups are completely avoided:

The Balanced Balanced Body compass

The main food groups eliminated on the AIP include:

- Grains (including pseudo-grains like quinoa)

- Legumes (beans, peanuts, soy, etc.)

- Dairy

- Eggs

- Nuts and seeds

- Nightshade vegetables (tomatoes, peppers, eggplant, etc.)

- Refined sugars and sweeteners

- Oils that may be inflammatory (corn, soy, canola, etc.)

- Alcohol

The Balanced Balanced Body compass

- NSAIDs like ibuprofen

- Food additives and preservatives

Allowable nutrient-dense, anti-inflammatory whole foods

- Vegetables (except nightshades)

- Fruit in moderation

- Quality proteins (grass-fed meat, wild-caught fish, etc.)

- Healthy fats (avocado, olive oil, coconut oil, etc.)

- Bone broth

- Safe spices and herbs

The Balanced Balanced Body compass

Healing the Gut

The process of healing leaky gut on the AIP encompasses the four Rs:

- Remove

  The first step is removing inflammatory foods, infections, and anything else that may be causing intestinal permeability and immune dysregulation.

- Replace

  Replace nutrients that are lacking by eating nutrient-dense whole foods and potentially supplementing with digestive enzymes, hydrochloric acid, etc.

- Reinoculate

  Reintroduce beneficial gut bacteria through probiotic-rich foods like ferments and potentially probiotic supplements.

The Balanced Balanced Body compass

- Repair

  Focus on foods and nutrients that help rebuild the gut lining barrier, including bone broth, L-glutamine, zinc, and healthy fats.

Reintroduction Protocol

To properly test each food group, follow this procedure:

1. Completely eliminate the food group for 2-4 weeks prior
2. Eat a generous portion of that single food over 2-3 days
3. Closely monitor for any returning symptoms over 4-7 days
4. If no reaction, that food can likely be incorporated back

The Balanced Balanced Body compass

5. If a reaction occurs, strictly remove that food group again

Potential Outcomes

1) Little to no reactivity - You're able to successfully add back most/all food groups and settle on a nutrient-dense, well-rounded diet.

2) Reactivity to some foods - You identify certain foods that seem to trigger symptoms and should be avoided or limited long-term.

3) Pervasive reactivity - If you react to nearly all foods reintroduced, it may indicate a need to continue on a very strict elimination diet a while longer before trying reintroductions again.

The Balanced Balanced Body compass

Chapter 1

RECIPE

SECTIONS

The Balanced Balanced Body compass

Quick and Easy Anti-Inflammatory Breakfast Recipes

1. Buffalo Ranch Breakfast Patties

Prep Time: 10 minutes
Cook Time: 15 minutes
Total Time: 25 minutes
Servings: 8 patties

Ingredients:

- 1 lb ground chicken or turkey
- 1 egg
- 1/4 cup buffalo sauce
- 2 tbsp ranch seasoning
- 1/4 cup green onions, sliced
- 1 tsp salt
- Avocado oil for cooking

Nutritional Value Per Patty:

The Balanced Balanced Body compass

Calories: 109,Fat: 6g,Carbs: 1g ,Fiber: 0gProtein: 12g

Instructions:

1. In a bowl, mix together the ground meat, egg, buffalo sauce, ranch seasoning, green onions and salt until fully combined.
2. Form mixture into 8 equal patties.
3. Heat avocado oil in a skillet over medium heat. Cook patties for 4-5 minutes per side until cooked through.
4. Serve warm with approved toppings like guacamole or salsa.

2. Sweet Potato Cauliflower Hash

Prep Time: 10 minutes
Cook Time: 20 minutes
Total Time: 30 minutes
Servings: 4

Ingredients:

- 1 medium sweet potato, diced

The Balanced Balanced Body compass

- 1 cup riced cauliflower
- 1/2 onion, diced
- 2 cloves garlic, minced
- 2 cups spinach, chopped
- 4 chicken sausage links, sliced
- 2 tbsp avocado oil
- 1 tsp dried thyme
- Salt and pepper to taste

Nutritional Value Per Serving:

Calories: 226 ,Fat: 13g,Carbs: 19g,Fiber: 5gProtein: 11g

Instructions:

1. Heat the oil in a skillet over medium heat. Add the diced sweet potato and cook for 5 minutes.
2. Add the onion and garlic and cook 2 more minutes.
3. Stir in the riced cauliflower, spinach, sausage, thyme and seasonings.
4. Continue cooking for 8-10 more minutes, stirring frequently, until vegetables are tender.
5. Adjust seasoning as needed before serving.

The Balanced Balanced Body compass

3. Banana Nut Muffins

Prep Time: 10 minutes
Cook Time: 25 minutes
Total Time: 35 minutes
Servings: 12 muffins

Ingredients:

- 1 1/4 cups coconut flour
- 1/2 cup arrowroot flour
- 1 tsp baking soda
- 1/2 tsp salt
- 3 eggs
- 1/4 cup maple syrup
- 1/4 cup coconut oil, melted
- 1 tsp vanilla
- 1/2 cup mashed ripe banana (about 1 large banana)
- 1/2 cup mixed nuts, chopped

Nutritional Value Per Muffin:
Calories: 193,Fat: 12g,Carbs: 18g,Fiber: 5g,Protein: 4g

Instructions:

1. Preheat oven to 350°F and line a muffin tin with liners.
2. In a large bowl, whisk the coconut flour, arrowroot, baking soda and salt.
3. In another bowl, mix the eggs, maple syrup, melted coconut oil, vanilla and banana.
4. Pour the wet ingredients into the dry and fold in with a spatula until just combined.
5. Fold in the chopped nuts.
6. Divide batter evenly among muffin cups.
7. Bake for 22-25 minutes until a toothpick inserted comes out clean.

4. Overnight Pumpkin Pie Oats

Prep Time: 5 minutes (+8 hrs to soak)
Cook Time: 0 minutes
Total Time: 8 hrs 5 minutes
Servings: 2

Ingredients:

The Balanced Balanced Body compass

- 1/2 cup coconut milk
- 1/2 cup pumpkin puree
- 2 tbsp maple syrup
- 1 tsp pumpkin pie spice
- 1/2 cup coconut yogurt
- 1/4 cup pumpkin seeds
- 1/2 cup mixed seeds (like sunflower, flax, chia)

Nutritional Value Per Serving:

Calories: 388 ,Fat: 25g,Carbs: 33g,Fiber: 10g,Protein: 14g

Instructions:

1. In a bowl, mix together the coconut milk, pumpkin, maple syrup and spices. Stir well.
2. Mix in the seeds and let soak covered in the fridge for at least 8 hours.
3. In the morning, stir in the coconut yogurt.
4. Top with extra pumpkin seeds, cinnamon or fruit if desired.

5. Carrot Cake Smoothie

Prep Time: 5 minutes
Cook Time: 0 minutes
Total Time: 5 minutes
Servings: 2

Ingredients:

- 1 cup coconut milk
- 1 frozen banana
- 1 cup carrots, chopped
- 1/2 cup pineapple chunks
- 2 tbsp coconut butter
- 1 tsp vanilla extract
- 1 tsp cinnamon
- 1/4 tsp nutmeg

Nutritional Value Per Serving:

Calories: 296,Fat: 22g,Carbs: 28g,Fiber: 6g,Protein: 4g

Instructions:

The Balanced Balanced Body compass

1. Add all ingredients to a blender and blend until completely smooth.
2. Add extra coconut milk to thin if needed.
3. Pour into glasses and optionally top with coconut flakes, nuts or seeds.

Overnight oats, smoothies, egg dishes, etc.

1. Tropical Smoothie Bowl
Prep Time: 5 minutes
Total Time: 5 minutes
Servings: 1

Ingredients:
- 1 frozen banana
- 1/2 cup frozen mango chunks
- 1/2 cup coconut milk
- 1 tbsp fresh lime juice
- 1 tbsp shredded unsweetened coconut
- 1 tbsp pomegranate seeds

Nutritional Value Per Serving:

The Balanced Balanced Body compass

Calories: 275,Fat: 10g,Carbs: 47g,Fiber: 6g
Protein: 2g

Instructions:

1. Blend frozen banana, mango, coconut milk and lime juice until smooth and thick.
2. Transfer to a bowl and top with shredded coconut and pomegranate seeds.

2. Tomato Basil Baked Eggs
Prep Time: 5 minutes
Cook Time: 15 minutes
Total Time: 20 minutes
Servings: 2

Ingredients:

- 4 eggs
- 1/2 cup cherry tomatoes, halved
- 2 tbsp fresh basil, chopped
- 1 tbsp olive oil
- Salt and pepper to taste

Nutritional Value Per Serving

The Balanced Balanced Body compass

Calories: 214,Fat: 17g,Carbs: 4g,Fiber: 1g,Protein: 13g

Instructions:

1. Preheat oven to 400°F.
2. Grease two ramekins and place them on a baking sheet.
3. Divide the tomatoes between the ramekins.
4. Crack 2 eggs into each ramekin on top of the tomatoes.
5. Drizzle with olive oil and season with salt, pepper and basil.
6. Bake for 12-15 minutes until egg whites are set.

3. Cinnamon Raisin Breakfast Flax Porridge
Prep Time: 5 minutes (+ soak time)
Cook Time: 0 minutes
Total Time: 8 hours 5 minutes
Servings: 2

Ingredients:

- 1/2 cup ground flaxseed
- 1 cup unsweetened almond milk
- 1/2 cup raisins

The Balanced Balanced Body compass

- 1 tsp cinnamon
- 1 tbsp maple syrup
- 2 tbsp chopped walnuts

Nutritional Value Per Serving:

Calories: 317,Fat: 14g,Carbs: 40g ,Fiber: 11g
Protein: 7g

Instructions:

1. In a bowl, mix together the ground flaxseed and almond milk. Cover and refrigerate for at least 8 hours.
2. In the morning, stir in the raisins, cinnamon and maple syrup.
3. Portion into bowls and top with chopped walnuts.

4. Paleo Breakfast Sausage Patties
Prep Time: 10 minutes
Cook Time: 10 minutes
Total Time: 20 minutes
Servings: 8 patties

The Balanced Balanced Body compass

Ingredients:

- 1 lb ground pork
- 1 tsp sage
- 1 tsp thyme
- 1/2 tsp salt
- 1/4 tsp black pepper
- 1/4 tsp red pepper flakes
- 2 cloves garlic, minced

Nutritional Value Per 2 Patties:

Calories: 229,Fat: 17g,Carbs: 1g,Fiber: 0g
Protein: 18g

Instructions:

1. In a bowl, mix together all ingredients until well combined.
2. Form into 8 equal patties.
3. Cook patties in a skillet over medium heat for 4-5 minutes per side until cooked through.
4. Serve warm alongside other breakfast dishes.

5. Coconut Flour Banana Pancakes

The Balanced Balanced Body compass

Prep Time: 5 minutes
Cook Time: 10 minutes
Total Time: 15 minutes
Servings: 2 (makes 6 pancakes)

Ingredients:

- 2 eggs
- 1 ripe banana, mashed
- 2 tbsp coconut flour
- 1 tsp baking powder
- 1/2 tsp cinnamon
- 1 tbsp coconut oil (for cooking)
- Toppings: fruit, nuts, maple syrup

Nutritional Value Per 3 Pancakes:

Calories: 204,Fat: 10g,Carbs: 24g,Fiber: 5g
Protein: 7g

Instructions:

1. In a bowl, whisk the eggs and mashed banana until combined.
2. Add in the coconut flour, baking powder and cinnamon. Mix well.

The Balanced Balanced Body compass

3. Heat coconut oil in a skillet over medium heat.
4. Pour batter into the skillet to form pancakes, about 3-inches across.
5. Cook 2-3 minutes per side until golden brown.
6. Serve warm with approved toppings like fresh fruit, nuts, and maple syrup.

Make-ahead breakfast meal prep ideas

1. Sweet Potato Toast Meal Prep

Prep Time: 15 mins
Cook Time: 45 mins
Total Time: 1 hr
Servings: 8 toasts

Ingredients:

- 2 large sweet potatoes, sliced 1/4-inch thick
- Toppings: mashed avocado, eggs, nut butter, seeds, etc.

The Balanced Balanced Body compass

Nutritional Value Per Toast (just sweet potato):

Calories: 105,Fat: 0g ,Carbs: 24g,Fiber: 3g
Protein: 2g

Instructions:

1. Preheat oven to 400°F. Line two baking sheets with parchment.
2. Arrange sweet potato slices on sheets.
3. Bake for 20 mins, then flip and bake 20 more mins until tender.
4. Let cool completely then store toasts in an airtight container.
5. In the morning, reheat and top with desired fixings.

2. Grain-Free Granola Bars

Prep Time: 10 mins
Cook Time: 25 mins
Total Time: 35 mins
Servings: 12 bars

The Balanced Balanced Body compass

Ingredients:

- 1 cup sunflower seed butter
- 1/2 cup coconut oil
- 1/3 cup maple syrup
- 1 tsp vanilla
- 1 cup unsweetened shredded coconut
- 1/2 cup pumpkin seeds
- 1/4 cup flaxseeds
- 1/3 cup dried fruit

Nutritional Value Per Bar:

Calories: 301 ,Fat: 24g,Carbs: 15g,Fiber: 4g
Protein: 7g

Instructions:

1. Preheat oven to 325°F. Line an 8x8 inch pan with parchment.
2. In a bowl, mix seed butter, coconut oil, syrup and vanilla.
3. Stir in coconut, seeds, flax and dried fruit until fully combined.
4. Press mixture evenly into prepared pan.
5. Bake for 22-25 minutes until lightly browned.

The Balanced Balanced Body compass

6. Let cool completely before cutting into 12 bars.

3. Breakfast Sausage Egg Cups

Prep Time: 15 mins
Cook Time: 20 mins
Total Time: 35 mins
Servings: 12 muffin cups

Ingredients:

- 1 lb ground chicken or turkey
- 1 tsp sage
- 1 tsp thyme
- 1/2 tsp salt
- 1/4 tsp black pepper
- 12 eggs
- 1/4 cup unsweetened almond milk
- 1/2 cup diced bell pepper

Nutritional Value Per Cup:

Calories: 150,Fat: 9g,Carbs: 1g,Fiber: 0g,
Protein: 14g

The Balanced Balanced Body compass

Instructions:

1. Preheat oven to 350°F. Grease a 12-cup muffin tin.
2. In a bowl, mix sausage ingredients until combined. Form into 12 balls.
3. Place one sausage ball in each muffin cup.
4. Whisk eggs and milk. Pour evenly over sausage balls.
5. Top with bell pepper.
6. Bake for 18-20 minutes until set.
7. Let cool before removing from tin. Refrigerate for up to 5 days.

4. Protein Breakfast Boxes

Prep Time: 20 mins
Total Time: 20 mins
Servings: 5 boxes

Ingredients:

- 5 hard-boiled eggs, peeled
- 1 cup grapes
- 5 oz cubed chicken or turkey
- 1 cup cucumber slices

The Balanced Balanced Body compass

- 1/4 cup nuts or seeds
- Guacamole or salsa for dipping (optional)

Nutritional Value Per Box:

Calories: 341,Fat: 18g,Carbs: 18g,Fiber: 4g
Protein: 27g

Instructions:

1. Hard boil the eggs and let cool completely before peeling.
2. Divide all the ingredients evenly into 5 portable containers with lids.
3. Store containers in the fridge for up to 4 days.
4. Grab and go in the morning!

5. Breakfast Protein Smoothie Packs

Prep Time: 10 mins
Total Time: 10 mins
Servings: 5 packs

Ingredients:

The Balanced Balanced Body compass

- 2 1/2 cups frozen cauliflower florets
- 2 cups frozen mango chunks
- 2 bananas, sliced and frozen
- 1/2 cup hemp seeds
- 1 tbsp ground flaxseed
- 1 tbsp nut or seed butter

Nutritional Value Per Pack:

Calories:285,Fat: 14g,Carbs: 32g,
Fiber: 9g ,Protein: 11g

Instructions:

1. Divide all the ingredients evenly into 5 ziplock bags or containers.
2. Store packs in the freezer for up to 1 month.
3. When ready, blend pack contents with 1 cup unsweetened milk.

11. Vegetable Frittata Muffins
Prep Time: 15 mins
Cook Time: 25 mins
Total Time: 40 mins
Servings: 12 muffins

Ingredients:

- 10 eggs
- 1/2 cup unsweetened almond milk
- 1 cup finely diced vegetables (bell pepper, spinach, zucchini, etc.)
- 1/4 cup diced onion
- 2 cloves garlic, minced
- 1 tsp dried basil
- 1/2 tsp salt

Nutritional Value Per Muffin:

Calories: 75,Fat: 5g,Carbs: 1g,Fiber: 0g
Protein: 6g

Instructions:

1. Preheat oven to 375°F and grease a 12-cup muffin tin.
2. In a bowl, whisk together eggs and milk.
3. Stir in vegetables, onion, garlic and seasonings.
4. Divide evenly into muffin cups.
5. Bake for 22-25 minutes until set in the center.
6. Let cool then refrigerate for up to 5 days.

The Balanced Balanced Body compass

vegetarian and vegan AIP (Autoimmune Protocol) friendly breakfast options:

1. Banana Coconut Chia Pudding
Prep Time: 5 minutes (+ 8 hours to set)
Total Time: 8 hours 5 minutes
Servings: 2

Ingredients:

- 1 ripe banana, mashed
- 1 1/4 cups coconut milk
- 1/4 cup chia seeds
- 1 tsp vanilla extract
- 1 tbsp maple syrup (optional)
- 2 tbsp unsweetened shredded coconut

Nutritional Value Per Serving:

The Balanced Balanced Body compass

Calories: 327,Fat: 18g,Carbs: 36g,Fiber: 14g
Protein: 7g

Instructions

1. In a bowl or jar, mix the mashed banana with coconut milk, chia seeds and vanilla.
2. Cover and refrigerate for at least 8 hours to thicken.
3. Stir in maple syrup if using.
4. Portion into bowls and top with shredded coconut.

2. Raspberry Coconut Flour Muffins
Prep Time: 10 minutes
Cook Time: 20 minutes
Total Time: 30 minutes
Servings: 8 muffins

Ingredients:

- 1/2 cup coconut flour
- 1/2 tsp baking soda
- 1/4 tsp salt
- 4 eggs
- 1/4 cup coconut oil, melted
- 1/4 cup maple syrup
- 1 tsp vanilla extract

The Balanced Balanced Body compass

- 1 cup fresh raspberries

Nutritional Value Per Muffin:

Calories: 161,Fat: 11g,Carbs: 12g,Fiber: 4g
Protein: 4g

Instructions:

1. Preheat oven to 350°F and line a muffin tin.
2. In a bowl, whisk the coconut flour, baking soda and salt.
3. In another bowl, whisk the eggs, then stir in coconut oil, maple syrup and vanilla.
4. Pour the wet into the dry and mix until fully combined.
5. Gently fold in the raspberries.
6. Scoop batter evenly into muffin cups.
7. Bake for 18-20 minutes until a toothpick inserted comes out clean.

3. Green Dream Smoothie
Prep Time: 5 minutes
Total Time: 5 minutes
Servings: 1

The Balanced Balanced Body compass

Ingredients:

- 1 banana
- 1 cup coconut milk
- 1 cup spinach
- 1/2 avocado
- 1 tbsp fresh grated ginger
- 1 tbsp chia seeds or flaxseeds

Nutritional Value Per Serving:

Calories: 431,Fat: 27g,Carbs: 47g,Fiber: 15g
Protein: 6g

Instructions:

1. Add all ingredients to a blender.
2. Blend until completely smooth and creamy.
3. Pour into a glass and enjoy!

4. Carrot Cake Baked Oatmeal Cups
Prep Time: 15 minutes
Cook Time: 25 minutes
Total Time: 40 minutes
Servings: 12 cups

Ingredients:

- 2 cups shredded carrots
- 1 cup coconut milk
- 1/2 cup applesauce
- 1/4 cup maple syrup
- 2 flax eggs (2 tbsp ground flaxseed + 6 tbsp water)
- 1 tsp vanilla extract
- 1 tsp cinnamon
- 1/2 tsp ginger
- 1/4 tsp nutmeg
- 1/4 tsp salt
- 1 cup coconut flour
- 1 tsp baking soda
- 1/2 cup raisins or chopped dates

Nutritional Value Per Cup:

Calories: 131,Fat: 5g,Carbs: 20g,Fiber: 4g
Protein: 2g

Instructions:

1. Preheat oven to 350°F and grease a 12-cup muffin tin.

2. Make flax eggs by mixing flaxseed and water. Let thicken for 5 mins.

3. In a bowl, mix shredded carrots, coconut milk, applesauce, maple syrup, flax eggs, vanilla and spices.

4. In another bowl, whisk the coconut flour, baking soda and salt.

5. Pour wet ingredients into dry and fold in raisins/dates until just combined.

6. Scoop batter evenly into muffin cups and bake for 22-25 minutes.

7. Let cool completely before removing from tin.

5. Coconut Yogurt Breakfast Bowls
Prep Time: 5 minutes
Total Time: 5 minutes
Servings: 2

Ingredients:

- 1 cup coconut yogurt
- 1 banana, sliced
- 1/2 cup fresh berries
- 2 tbsp granola (grain-free)

The Balanced Balanced Body compass

- 2 tbsp nut or seed butter
- 1 tbsp chia seeds
- Drizzle of maple syrup

Nutritional Value Per Serving:

Calories: 424,Fat: 26g,Carbs: 40g,Fiber: 12g
Protein: 9g

Instructions:

1. In a bowl or jar, layer half of the coconut yogurt.
2. Top with half of the banana slices, berries, granola, nut butter, chia seeds and maple syrup.
3. Repeat layers in a second bowl/jar.

plant-based main dish recipes that are AIP-compliant:

1. Loaded Sweet Potato
Prep Time: 10 minutes
Cook Time: 60 minutes

The Balanced Balanced Body compass

Total Time: 1 hour 10 minutes
Servings: 4

Ingredients:

- 4 medium sweet potatoes
- 1 cup sautéed spinach
- 1/2 cup diced tomatoes
- 1/4 cup diced onion
- 2 tbsp coconut butter
- 1/4 cup coconut yogurt
- 1 tsp garlic powder
- 1 tsp onion powder
- 1/4 tsp salt

Nutritional Value Per Serving:

Calories: 256,Fat: 8g,Carbs: 41g,Fiber: 7g
Protein: 4g

Instructions:

1. Preheat oven to 400°F. Prick sweet potatoes with a fork and bake for 50-60 minutes until very soft.
2. In a skillet, sauté the spinach, tomatoes and onion for 5 minutes until heated through.

The Balanced Balanced Body compass

3. Let sweet potatoes cool slightly, then slice open. Use a fork to mash insides slightly.

4. Top each sweet potato half with sautéed veggies, coconut butter, yogurt and seasonings.

2. Spaghetti Squash with Pesto
Prep Time: 10 minutes
Cook Time: 45 minutes
Total Time: 55 minutes
Servings: 4

Ingredients:

For the Squash:
- 1 medium spaghetti squash, halved lengthwise and seeded

For the Pesto:
- 2 cups fresh basil leaves
- 1/4 cup pine nuts
- 3 cloves garlic
- 1/3 cup olive oil
- 2 tbsp lemon juice
- 1/2 tsp salt

Nutritional Value Per Serving:

The Balanced Balanced Body compass

Calories: 328,Fat: 27g,Carbs: 20g,Fiber: 4g
Protein: 6g

Instructions:

1. Preheat oven to 400°F. Place squash halves cut-side down on a baking sheet and bake for 40 minutes.
2. Meanwhile, make the pesto by blitzing all pesto ingredients in a food processor until combined.
3. Once squash is tender when pierced with a fork, use a fork to scrape the flesh into spaghetti-like strands.
4. Toss the spaghetti squash strands with the fresh pesto until fully coated. Serve warm.

3. Cauliflower Rice Burrito Bowls
Prep Time: 20 minutes
Cook Time: 10 minutes
Total Time: 30 minutes
Servings: 4

Ingredients:

The Balanced Balanced Body compass

- 1 head cauliflower, riced
- 1 cup diced tomatoes
- 1 cup diced bell peppers
- 1/2 cup diced onion
- 1 (15 oz) can pumpkin puree
- 2 tsp chili powder
- 1 tsp ground cumin
- 1 tsp garlic powder
- 1/2 tsp salt
- Toppings: diced avocado, shredded lettuce, lime wedges

Nutritional Value Per Serving:

Calories: 155,Fat: 4g,Carbs: 25g,Fiber: 9g
Protein: 6g

Instructions:

1. In a skillet, sauté the diced tomatoes, peppers and onion for 5 minutes.
2. Add the riced cauliflower and spices. Cook for 3 more minutes.
3. Remove from heat and stir in the pumpkin puree until well combined.

4. Serve burrito bowl-style in bowls topped with avocado, shredded lettuce and lime wedges.

4. Baked Vegetable Cakes
Prep Time: 20 minutes
Cook Time: 25 minutes
Total Time: 45 minutes
Servings: 6 cakes

Ingredients:

- 1 cup shredded zucchini
- 1 cup shredded carrots
- 1 cup shredded beets
- 1 cup shredded plantain or green banana
- 3 eggs, beaten
- 1/4 cup coconut flour
- 1 tsp baking powder
- 1/2 tsp salt
- 1/4 tsp garlic powder
- 1/4 cup coconut oil, melted

Nutritional Value Per Cake:

Calories: 196,Fat: 12g,Carbs: 20g ,Fiber: 4g
Protein: 4g

The Balanced Balanced Body compass

Instructions:

1. Preheat oven to 375°F and grease a baking sheet.
2. In a large bowl, mix together all shredded vegetables.
3. In a separate bowl, whisk the eggs, then mix in coconut flour, baking powder, salt and garlic powder.
4. Pour the coconut oil into the dry ingredients and mix well.
5. Fold the wet ingredients into the shredded vegetables until fully combined.
6. Scoop batter into 6 mounds on the baking sheet. Flatten into rounds.
7. Bake for 22-25 minutes until lightly browned.
8. Serve warm with your choice of AIP-friendly toppings.

5. Moroccan Stuffed Spaghetti Squash
Prep Time: 15 minutes
Cook Time: 1 hour
Total Time: 1 hour 15 minutes
Servings: 4

Ingredients:

The Balanced Balanced Body compass

- 1 medium spaghetti squash, halved lengthwise and seeded
- 2 cups finely chopped kale
- 1 cup diced carrots
- 1/2 cup raisins
- 1/4 cup pine nuts
- 2 cloves garlic, minced
- 1 tsp ground cumin
- 1 tsp ground cinnamon
- 1/2 tsp salt
- 1/4 cup coconut butter, melted

Nutritional Value Per Serving:

Calories: 322,Fat: 19g,Carbs: 40g,Fiber: 8g
Protein: 6g

Instructions:

1. Preheat oven to 400°F. Place squash halves cut-side down on a baking sheet. Roast for 40-45 mins.
2. In a skillet, sauté the kale, carrots, raisins, pine nuts, garlic and spices for 5 minutes.
3. When squash is tender, use a fork to scrape the flesh into strands.

4. Toss the squash strands with the veggie filling and melted coconut butter until fully coated.

5. Stuff the squash halves with the filling mixture and serve warm.

legume-based dishes that follow the AIP diet:

1. White Bean and Artichoke Dip
Prep Time: 10 minutes
Cook Time: 0 minutes
Total Time: 10 minutes
Servings: 8 (1/4 cup each)

Ingredients:

- 1 (15oz) can white beans, rinsed and drained
- 1 (14oz) can artichoke hearts, drained
- 1/4 cup olive oil
- 2 cloves garlic
- 2 tbsp lemon juice
- 1 tsp dried basil
- 1/2 tsp salt

Nutritional Value Per Serving:

Calories: 126,Fat: 8g,Carbs: 11g,Fiber: 4g
Protein: 4g

Instructions:

1. Add all ingredients to a food processor or blender.
2. Process until smooth and creamy, scraping down sides as needed.
3. Transfer to a serving bowl and serve with veggie sticks or plantain chips.

2. Chickpea Curry
Prep Time: 15 minutes
Cook Time: 30 minutes
Total Time: 45 minutes
Servings: 4

Ingredients:

- 1 tbsp coconut oil
- 1 onion, diced
- 3 cloves garlic, minced

The Balanced Balanced Body compass

- 1 tbsp grated ginger
- 2 tsp curry powder
- 1 tsp garam masala
- 1 (15oz) can diced tomatoes
- 1 (15oz) can chickpeas, drained and rinsed
- 1 cup coconut milk
- 1 cup vegetable broth
- 1/2 tsp salt
- Chopped cilantro for serving

Nutritional Value Per Serving

Calories: 384,Fat: 21g,Carbs: 43g,Fiber: 12g
Protein: 11g

Instructions:

1. In a skillet, heat the coconut oil over medium heat.
2. Add the onion and sauté for 5 minutes until translucent.
3. Stir in the garlic, ginger and spices and cook for 1 minute.
4. Pour in the tomatoes, chickpeas, coconut milk, broth and salt.
5. Bring to a simmer and cook for 15-20 minutes.

6. Garnish with cilantro before serving over cauliflower rice.

3. Lentil Sloppy Joes
Prep Time: 10 minutes
Cook Time: 25 minutes
Total Time: 35 minutes
Servings: 4

Ingredients:

- 1 tbsp coconut oil
- 1 onion, diced
- 2 cloves garlic, minced
- 1 cup dried brown lentils, rinsed
- 1 cup vegetable broth
- 1 (6oz) can tomato paste
- 2 tbsp coconut aminos
- 1 tbsp apple cider vinegar
- 1 tsp yellow mustard powder
- 1/2 tsp salt
- 1/4 tsp black pepper

Lettuce leaves or sweet potato buns for serving

Nutritional Value Per Serving (lentil mixture only):

The Balanced Balanced Body compass

Calories: 229,Fat: 3g,Carbs: 38g,Fiber: 15g,Protein: 14g

Instructions:

1. In a skillet, heat the coconut oil over medium heat.
2. Sauté the onion for 5 minutes until translucent. Add the garlic and cook 1 minute more.
3. Stir in the lentils, broth, tomato paste, aminos, vinegar, mustard and spices.
4. Bring to a simmer and cook for 20 minutes, until lentils are very soft, mashing some with a fork.
5. Serve lentil mixture over lettuce leaves or sweet potato buns.

4. Split Pea Soup
Prep Time: 10 minutes
Cook Time: 60 minutes
Total Time: 1 hour 10 minutes
Servings: 6

Ingredients:

- 1 tbsp olive oil
- 1 onion, diced

The Balanced Balanced Body compass

- 3 carrots, diced
- 3 stalks celery, diced
- 3 cloves garlic, minced
- 1 lb dried split green peas, rinsed
- 6 cups vegetable broth
- 2 bay leaves
- 1 tsp dried thyme
- 1/2 tsp black pepper

Nutritional Value Per Serving:

Calories: 234,Fat: 4g,Carbs: 38g,Fiber: 16g,Protein: 14g

Instructions:

1. In a large pot, heat the olive oil over medium heat.
2. Add the onion, carrots and celery. Sauté for 5-7 minutes until softened.
3. Stir in the garlic and cook 1 minute more.
4. Add the split peas, broth, bay leaves, thyme and pepper.
5. Bring to a boil, then reduce heat and simmer for 45-60 minutes, until peas are very soft.

6. Remove bay leaves before serving. Use an immersion blender to partially puree for a creamy texture if desired.

5. Nutty Lentil Loaf
Prep Time: 20 minutes
Cook Time: 60 minutes
Total Time: 1 hour 20 minutes
Servings: 8 slices

Ingredients:

- 1 cup dried green lentils
- 1 1/2 cups vegetable broth
- 1 onion, diced
- 2 carrots, grated
- 1 cup grated zucchini
- 1 cup finely chopped pecans or walnuts
- 2 eggs, beaten
- 1/2 cup coconut flour
- 1 tbsp coconut aminos
- 1 tsp dried thyme
- 1 tsp garlic powder
- 1/2 tsp salt

Nutritional Value Per Slice:

The Balanced Balanced Body compass

Calories: 251,Fat: 14g,Carbs: 24g ,Fiber: 8g,Protein: 9g

Instructions:

1. Cook lentils in broth according to package instructions. Drain excess liquid if needed.
2. Preheat oven to 375°F and grease a loaf pan.
3. In a bowl, mash half the cooked lentils. Mix in remaining whole lentils.
4. Stir in onion, carrots, zucchini, nuts, eggs, coconut flour, aminos, and seasonings until fully combined.
5. Press mixture firmly into prepared loaf pan.
6. Bake for 50-60 minutes until set.
7. Let cool 10 minutes before slicing.

grain-free vegetarian recipe

1. Zucchini Noodles with Creamy Avocado Pesto

Prep Time: 15 minutes
Cook Time: 5 minutes
Total Time: 20 minutes

The Balanced Balanced Body compass

Servings: 4

Ingredients:

- 4 medium zucchinis, spiralized or julienned
- 1 avocado
- 1 cup fresh basil leaves
- 1/4 cup pine nuts
- 2 cloves garlic, minced
- 2 tablespoons lemon juice
- 1/4 cup olive oil
- 1/4 teaspoon salt
- 1/4 teaspoon black pepper

Nutritional Information (per serving):

Calories: 270, Total Fat: 24g, Saturated Fat: 3g,Cholesterol: 0mg,Sodium: 150mg
Total Carbohydrates: 13g,Dietary Fiber: 5g,Protein: 5g

Instructions:

1. Spiralize or julienne the zucchinis and set aside.

2. In a food processor, combine the avocado, basil, pine nuts, garlic, lemon juice, olive oil, salt, and pepper. Process until smooth and creamy.

3. Toss the zucchini noodles with the avocado pesto sauce until well coated.

4. Serve immediately, garnished with extra basil leaves and pine nuts if desired.

2. Cauliflower Crust Pizza with Veggie Toppings

Prep Time: 20 minutes
Cook Time: 30 minutes
Total Time: 50 minutes
Servings: 4

Ingredients:

- 1 head cauliflower, grated or riced
- 2 eggs
- 1/2 cup almond flour
- 1/2 teaspoon salt
- 1/2 teaspoon Italian seasoning
- 1 cup marinara sauce
- 1 cup sliced mushrooms
- 1 bell pepper, sliced
- 1/2 red onion, sliced

The Balanced Balanced Body compass

- 1/2 cup sliced olives

Nutritional Information (per serving):

Calories: 230,Total Fat: 12g,Saturated Fat: 2g,Cholesterol: 95mg,Sodium: 690mg,
Total Carbohydrates: 22g,Dietary Fiber: 6g,Protein: 10g

Instructions:

1. Preheat your oven to 425°F (220°C).
2. In a large bowl, combine the grated cauliflower, eggs, almond flour, salt, and Italian seasoning. Mix well until a dough forms.
3. Press the cauliflower dough onto a parchment-lined baking sheet, forming a pizza crust shape.
4. Bake the cauliflower crust for 15 minutes.
5. Remove the crust from the oven and top with marinara sauce, sliced mushrooms, bell pepper, red onion, and olives.
6. Return the pizza to the oven and bake for an additional 10-15 minutes, or until the crust is golden brown and the toppings are cooked through.
7. Allow the pizza to cool slightly before slicing and serving.

The Balanced Balanced Body compass

3. Stuffed Portobello Mushrooms with Spinach and Feta

Prep Time: 15 minutes
Cook Time: 20 minutes
Total Time: 35 minutes
Servings: 4

Ingredients:

- 4 large portobello mushroom caps
- 2 cups fresh spinach leaves
- 1/2 cup crumbled feta cheese
- 2 cloves garlic, minced
- 2 tablespoons olive oil
- Salt and pepper to taste

nutritional information (per serving):

Calories: 180, Total Fat: 12g,Saturated Fat: 4g
Cholesterol: 20mg, Sodium: 390mgTotal
Carbohydrates: 10g,Dietary Fiber: 4g,Protein: 8g

Instructions:

The Balanced Balanced Body compass

1. Preheat your oven to 375°F (190°C).
2. Remove the stems from the portobello mushroom caps and use a spoon to gently scoop out the gills, creating a cavity for the stuffing.
3. In a bowl, mix together the spinach, feta cheese, minced garlic, olive oil, salt, and pepper.
4. Stuff the filling mixture into the portobello mushroom caps, distributing it evenly.
5. Place the stuffed mushrooms on a baking sheet lined with parchment paper.
6. Bake for 18-20 minutes, or until the mushrooms are tender and the filling is heated through.
7. Serve the stuffed portobello mushrooms warm.

4. Baked Sweet Potato Fries with Chipotle Lime Dip

Prep Time: 15 minutes
Cook Time: 25 minutes
Total Time: 40 minutes
Servings: 4

Ingredients:

- 4 medium sweet potatoes, cut into fry shapes
- 2 tablespoons olive oil

The Balanced Balanced Body compass

- 1 teaspoon paprika
- 1/2 teaspoon garlic powder
- 1/2 teaspoon salt

For the Chipotle Lime Dip:

- 1/2 cup cashew butter
- 1/4 cup water
- 2 tablespoons lime juice
- 1 chipotle pepper in adobo sauce
- 1/4 teaspoon salt

Nutritional Information (per serving):

Calories: 340,Total Fat: 18g,Saturated Fat: 3g,Cholesterol: 0mg,Sodium: 440mgTotal Carbohydrates: 43g,Dietary Fiber: 7g,Protein: 6g

Instructions:

1. Preheat your oven to 425°F (220°C).
2. In a large bowl, toss the cut sweet potato fries with olive oil, paprika, garlic powder, and salt until well coated.
3. Spread the sweet potato fries in a single layer on a baking sheet lined with parchment paper.

4. Bake for 20-25 minutes, flipping halfway through, until the fries are tender and crispy.

5. While the fries are baking, prepare the chipotle lime dip by blending all the dip ingredients in a food processor or blender until smooth.

6. Serve the baked sweet potato fries hot with the chipotle lime dip on the side for dipping.

Chicken , turkey, and beef recipes

1. Beef and Vegetable Stir-Fry

Prep Time: 20 minutes
Cook Time: 10 minutes
Total Time: 30 minutes
Servings: 4

Ingredients:

1 lb flank steak or sirloin, thinly sliced against the grain

2 tablespoons coconut or avocado oil

1 red bell pepper, sliced

1 cup broccoli florets

1 cup snap peas

The Balanced Balanced Body compass

1 cup sliced mushrooms

2 cloves garlic, minced

1 tablespoon grated fresh ginger

2 tablespoons coconut aminos or tamari sauce

1 tablespoon rice vinegar

Salt and pepper to taste

Sesame seeds for garnish

Nutritional Information (per serving):

Calories: 290,Total Fat: 14g, Saturated Fat: 5g
Cholesterol: 60mg,Sodium: 470mg,Total
Carbohydrates: 12g,Dietary Fiber: 3g,Protein: 28g

Instructions:

1. In a large skillet or wok, heat the coconut or avocado oil over high heat.

2. Add the sliced beef and stir-fry for 2-3 minutes until browned but not fully cooked.

3. Add the sliced bell pepper, broccoli florets, snap peas, sliced mushrooms, minced garlic, and grated ginger. Stir-fry for 3-4 minutes, or until the vegetables are tender-crisp.

4. Add the coconut aminos (or tamari sauce) and rice vinegar. Toss everything together and season with salt and pepper to taste.

5. Serve the stir-fry hot, garnished with sesame seeds if desired.

2. Baked Lemon Herb Turkey Meatballs

Prep Time: 20 minutes
Cook Time: 20 minutes
Total Time: 40 minutes
Servings: 4 (6 meatballs per serving)

Ingredients:

- 1 lb ground turkey
- 1 egg
- 1/2 cup almond flour
- 1/4 cup finely chopped parsley
- 2 tablespoons lemon juice
- 2 cloves garlic, minced
- 1 teaspoon dried oregano
- 1/2 teaspoon salt

The Balanced Balanced Body compass

- 1/4 teaspoon black pepper

Nutritional Information (per serving):

Calories: 260,Total Fat: 14g,Saturated Fat: 3g,Cholesterol: 125mg,Sodium: 480mg,Total Carbohydrates: 6g,Dietary Fiber: 2g,Protein: 27g

Instructions:

1. Preheat oven to 375°F (190°C). Line a baking sheet with parchment paper.
2. In a large bowl, combine ground turkey, egg, almond flour, parsley, lemon juice, garlic, oregano, salt, and pepper. Mix well until fully combined.
3. Form the mixture into 24 equal-sized meatballs and place them on the prepared baking sheet.
4. Bake for 18-20 minutes, or until the meatballs are cooked through and lightly browned on the outside.
5. Serve hot, with desired dipping sauce or over a bed of greens or zucchini noodles.

3. Beef and Mushroom Stuffed Peppers

Prep Time: 20 minutes
Cook Time: 40 minutes

The Balanced Balanced Body compass

Total Time: 1 hour
Servings: 4

Ingredients:

4 large bell peppers (any color), tops cut off and seeded
  1 lb ground beef
  1 cup sliced mushrooms
  1 onion, diced
  2 cloves garlic, minced
  1 (14.5 oz) can diced tomatoes
  1 teaspoon dried oregano
  1/2 teaspoon salt
  1/4 teaspoon black pepper

Nutritional Information (per serving):

Calories: 350,Total Fat: 18, Saturated Fat: 6g
 Cholesterol: 75mg,Sodium: 590mg,Total
Carbohydrates: 20g, Dietary Fiber: 5g, Protein: 28g

Instructions:

1. Preheat oven to 375°F (190°C).

The Balanced Balanced Body compass

2. In a skillet over medium-high heat, cook the ground beef until browned and crumbled. Drain excess fat.

3. Add the sliced mushrooms, diced onion, and minced garlic to the skillet. Cook for 3-4 minutes, until the onions are translucent.

4. Stir in the diced tomatoes, dried oregano, salt, and black pepper. Simmer for 5 minutes.

5. Stuff the beef and mushroom mixture into the hollowed-out bell peppers, packing it tightly.

6. Place the stuffed peppers in a baking dish and add a little water to the bottom of the dish to prevent burning.

7. Bake for 35-40 minutes, or until the peppers are tender and the filling is heated through.

8. Serve hot, garnished with fresh parsley or cilantro if desired.

4. Grilled Chicken Skewers with Pineapple Salsa

Prep Time: 20 minutes (plus 30 minutes marinating time)
Cook Time: 10-12 minutes
Total Time: 1 hour
Servings: 4

The Balanced Balanced Body compass

Ingredients:

For the Chicken Skewers:

- 1 1/2 lbs boneless, skinless chicken breasts, cut into 1-inch cubes
- 1/4 cup olive oil
- 2 tablespoons lime juice
- 2 cloves garlic, minced
- 1 teaspoon cumin
- 1 teaspoon chili powder
- 1/2 teaspoon salt
- 1/4 teaspoon black pepper

For the Pineapple Salsa:

- 1 cup diced fresh pineapple
- 1/4 cup diced red onion
- 1/4 cup chopped cilantro
- 1 jalapeño, seeded and finely chopped
- 2 tablespoons lime juice
- Salt and pepper to taste

Nutritional Information (per serving):

Calories: 320,Total Fat: 15g,Saturated Fat: 2g

The Balanced Balanced Body compass

Cholesterol: 110mg, Sodium: 460mg,
Total Carbohydrates: 14g,Dietary Fiber: 2g
Protein: 34g

Instructions:

1. In a shallow dish or resealable bag, combine the cubed chicken, olive oil, lime juice, minced garlic, cumin, chili powder, salt, and black pepper. Marinate for 30 minutes, or up to 2 hours in the refrigerator.
2. Meanwhile, prepare the pineapple salsa by combining the diced pineapple, red onion, cilantro, jalapeño, lime juice, and salt and pepper to taste. Set aside.
3. Preheat grill or grill pan to medium-high heat.
4. Thread the marinated chicken onto skewers, leaving a little space between each piece.
5. Grill the chicken skewers for 10-12 minutes, turning occasionally, until the chicken is cooked through and slightly charred.
6. Serve the grilled chicken skewers hot, with the pineapple salsa on the side for topping.

5. Beef and Vegetable Kabobs

The Balanced Balanced Body compass

Prep Time: 20 minutes (plus 30 minutes marinating time)
Cook Time: 12-15 minutes
Total Time: 1 hour
Servings: 4

Ingredients:

- 1 lb sirloin steak, cut into 1-inch cubes
- 1 red bell pepper, cut into 1-inch pieces
- 1 yellow squash, cut into 1-inch pieces
- 1 zucchini, cut into 1-inch pieces
- 1 red onion, cut into 1-inch pieces
- 1/4 cup olive oil
- 2 tablespoons balsamic vinegar
- 2 cloves garlic, minced
- 1 teaspoon dried oregano
- 1/2 teaspoon salt
- 1/4 teaspoon black pepper

Nutritional Information (per serving):

Calories: 380,Total Fat: 24g,Saturated Fat: 6g
Cholesterol: 60mg,Sodium: 380mg
Total Carbohydrates: 16g,Dietary Fiber: 3g
Protein: 26g

The Balanced Balanced Body compass

Instructions:

1. In a shallow dish or resealable bag, combine the cubed sirloin steak, bell pepper, yellow squash, zucchini, and red onion.
2. In a small bowl, whisk together the olive oil, balsamic vinegar, minced garlic, dried oregano, salt, and black pepper.
3. Pour the marinade over the steak and vegetable pieces, tossing to coat evenly. Marinate for 30 minutes, or up to 2 hours in the refrigerator.
4. Preheat grill or grill pan to medium-high heat.
5. Thread the marinated steak and vegetables onto skewers, alternating between the different ingredients.
6. Grill the kabobs for 12-15 minutes, turning occasionally, until the steak is cooked to your desired doneness and the vegetables are tender and lightly charred.
7. Serve the beef and vegetable kabobs hot, garnished with fresh parsley or cilantro if desired.

These recipes offer a variety of protein options from chicken, turkey, and beef, accompanied by flavorful seasonings and nutrient-dense vegetables. They are suitable

Poultry, meat, and potato dishes

1. Grilled Flank Steak with Loaded Baked Potatoes

Prep Time: 20 minutes (plus 30 minutes marinating time)
Cook Time: 30 minutes
Total Time: 1 hour 20 minutes
Servings: 4

Ingredients:

For the Flank Steak:
- 1 1/2 lbs flank steak
- 1/4 cup olive oil
- 2 tablespoons balsamic vinegar
- 2 cloves garlic, minced
- 1 teaspoon dried rosemary
- 1/2 teaspoon salt
- 1/4 teaspoon black pepper

The Balanced Balanced Body compass

For the Loaded Baked Potatoes:

- 4 large russet potatoes
- 4 tablespoons butter
- 1/2 cup full-fat coconut milk or dairy-free milk
- Salt and pepper to taste
- Chopped chives or green onions for garnish
- Bacon bits or crispy bacon (optional)

Nutritional Information (per serving):

Calories: 680,Total Fat: 36g,Saturated Fat: 14g
Cholesterol: 95mg,Sodium: 560mg
Total Carbohydrates: 51g,Dietary Fiber: 5g
Protein: 38g

Instructions:

1. In a shallow dish or resealable bag, combine the flank steak with olive oil, balsamic vinegar, minced garlic, dried rosemary, salt, and black pepper. Marinate for 30 minutes to 2 hours in the refrigerator.
2. Preheat your grill or grill pan to medium-high heat.

3. Prick the russet potatoes several times with a fork and place them on a baking sheet or directly on the oven rack. Bake at 400°F (200°C) for 1 hour or until tender when pierced with a fork.

4. Grill the marinated flank steak for 6-8 minutes per side, or until it reaches your desired doneness. Let it rest for 5 minutes before slicing against the grain.

5. Once the potatoes are done, slice them open and fluff the insides with a fork.

6. Add butter and coconut milk (or dairy-free milk) to the potatoes. Season with salt and pepper to taste.

7. Top the loaded baked potatoes with sliced grilled flank st

2. Chicken Fajita Bowls with Roasted Sweet Potatoes

Prep Time: 20 minutes
Cook Time: 30 minutes
Total Time: 50 minutes
Servings: 4

Ingredients:

- 1 lb boneless, skinless chicken breasts, sliced into strips
- 2 bell peppers (any color), sliced
- 1 red onion, sliced
- 2 tablespoons olive oil
- 1 tablespoon fajita seasoning
- 2 medium sweet potatoes, cubed
- 1 tablespoon olive oil
- Salt and pepper to taste
- Lime wedges for serving

Nutritional Information (per serving):

Calories: 370,Total Fat: 15g,Saturated Fat: 2g
Cholesterol: 65mg,Sodium: 290mg
Total Carbohydrates: 32g, Dietary Fiber: 6g
Protein: 28g

Instructions:

1. Preheat oven to 400°F (200°C).
2. On a baking sheet, toss the cubed sweet potatoes with 1 tablespoon olive oil, salt, and pepper. Roast for 25-30 minutes, until tender and lightly browned.
3. In a large skillet or grill pan, heat the remaining 2 tablespoons of olive oil over medium-high heat.

4. Add the sliced chicken, bell peppers, and red onion to the skillet. Sprinkle with fajita seasoning and sauté for 8-10 minutes, stirring occasionally, until chicken is cooked through and vegetables are tender.

5. To serve, divide the roasted sweet potatoes into bowls and top with the chicken fajita mixture.

6. Squeeze fresh lime juice over the top and serve with desired toppings like avocado, salsa, etc.

3. Pork Tenderloin with Rosemary Roasted Potatoes

Prep Time: 15 minutes
Cook Time: 45 minutes
Total Time: 1 hour
Servings: 4

Ingredients:

- 1 pork tenderloin (about 1 lb)
- 2 tablespoons olive oil, divided
- 1 teaspoon salt
- 1/2 teaspoon black pepper
- 1 lb baby potatoes, halved
- 2 tablespoons fresh rosemary, chopped
- 2 cloves garlic, minced

Nutritional Information (per serving):

- Calories: 410
Total Fat: 16g,Saturated Fat: 3g,Cholesterol: 95mg
Sodium: 720mg,Total Carbohydrates: 30g,Dietary
Fiber: 3g,Protein: 36g

Instructions:

1. Preheat oven to 400°F (200°C).
2. Pat the pork tenderloin dry and season all over with salt and pepper.
3. Heat 1 tablespoon olive oil in an oven-safe skillet over medium-high heat. Sear the pork on all sides until browned, about 2 minutes per side. Transfer to a plate.
4. In the same skillet, toss the halved baby potatoes with the remaining 1 tablespoon olive oil, chopped rosemary, and minced garlic until well coated.
5. Nestle the seared pork tenderloin in the center of the potatoes.
6. Roast in the preheated oven for 25-30 minutes, or until the pork reaches an internal temperature of 145°F (63°C) and the potatoes are tender and crispy.

The Balanced Balanced Body compass

7. Let the pork rest for 5 minutes before slicing and serving with the roasted potatoes.

4. Beef Kofta Kebabs with Roasted Potatoes

Prep Time: 25 minutes (plus 30 minutes chilling time)
Cook Time: 20 minutes
Total Time: 1 hour 15 minutes
Servings: 4

Ingredients:

For the Kofta:

- 1 lb ground beef
- 1/2 onion, finely chopped
- 3 cloves garlic, minced
- 1 teaspoon ground cumin
- 1 teaspoon ground coriander
- 1 teaspoon paprika
- 1/2 teaspoon salt
- 1/4 teaspoon black pepper

For the Potatoes:

- 1 lb small potatoes, quartered
- 2 tablespoons olive oil
- 1 teaspoon dried oregano
- Salt and pepper to taste

Nutritional Information (per serving):

Calories: 460,Total Fat: 25g
Saturated Fat: 8g,Cholesterol: 100mg
 Sodium: 540mg,Total Carbohydrates: 28g
Dietary Fiber: 3g,Protein: 31g

Instructions:

1. In a large bowl, mix together all the kofta ingredients until well combined. Cover and chill for 30 minutes to allow flavors to meld.
2. Preheat oven to 425°F (220°C).
3. On a baking sheet, toss the quartered potatoes with olive oil, dried oregano, salt, and pepper until evenly coated.
4. Roast the potatoes for 20-25 minutes, flipping halfway, until tender and golden brown.
5. Meanwhile, form the chilled kofta mixture into oval-shaped kebabs, about 6-8 per skewer.

6. Grill or broil the kofta kebabs for 8-10 minutes, turning occasionally, until cooked through.

7. Serve the kofta kebabs with the roasted potatoes, garnished with chopped parsley and tzatziki sauce if desired.

5. Herb Crusted Pork Chops with Garlic Mashed Potatoes

Prep Time: 15 minutes
Cook Time: 30 minutes
Total Time: 45 minutes
Servings: 4

Ingredients:

For the Pork Chops:
- 4 bone-in pork chops
- 2 tablespoons olive oil
- 1/2 cup panko breadcrumbs
- 1/4 cup grated Parmesan
- 2 tablespoons fresh parsley, chopped
- 1 teaspoon dried thyme
- 1/2 teaspoon salt
- 1/4 teaspoon black pepper

The Balanced Balanced Body compass

For the Mashed Potatoes:

- 2 lbs russet potatoes, peeled and cubed
- 4 tablespoons butter or ghee
- 1/2 cup unsweetened almond milk or broth
- 4 cloves garlic, minced
- Salt and pepper to taste

Nutritional Information (per serving):

Calories: 620,Total Fat: 30g,Saturated Fat: 12g
Cholesterol: 125mg, Sodium: 870mg
Total Carbohydrates: 51g,Dietary Fiber: 5g
 Protein: 37g

Instructions:

1. Preheat oven to 400°F (200°C).
2. In a shallow bowl, mix together the panko breadcrumbs, Parmesan, parsley, thyme, salt, and pepper.
3. Brush the pork chops with olive oil on both sides, then dredge in the breadcrumb mixture, pressing to adhere.

4. Place the breaded pork chops on a baking sheet and bake for 20-25 minutes until golden brown and cooked through.

5. Meanwhile, boil the cubed potatoes until tender, about 15 minutes. Drain well.

6. Return the potatoes to the pot and mash with butter, almond milk, and minced garlic until smooth and creamy. Season with salt and pepper.

7. Serve the herb-crusted pork chops hot with the garlic mashed potatoes on the side.

These poultry, meat and potato dishes offer a variety of flavors and cooking methods, from roasted and grilled to skillet meals. They provide complete protein sources along with nutrient-dense vegetables and starches in a satisfying way.

seafood entrees

1. Baked Salmon with Lemon Dill Sauce

Prep Time: 10 minutes
Cook Time: 15 minutes
Total Time: 25 minutes

Servings: 4

Ingredients:

- 4 (6 oz) salmon fillets
- Salt and pepper to taste
- 2 tablespoons olive oil
- 2 tablespoons butter
- 2 cloves garlic, minced
- 2 tablespoons lemon juice
- 2 tablespoons chopped fresh dill
- 1/4 cup dry white wine or broth

Nutritional Information (per serving):

Calories: 350
Total Fat: 22g,Saturated Fat: 5g,Cholesterol: 95mg
Sodium: 200mg,Total Carbohydrates: 2g
Dietary Fiber: 0g,Protein: 34g

Instructions:

1. Preheat oven to 400°F (200°C).
2. Season salmon fillets with salt and pepper.
3. Heat olive oil in an oven-safe skillet over medium-high heat.

The Balanced Balanced Body compass

4. Sear salmon fillets for 2 minutes per side until lightly browned.

5. Transfer skillet to the preheated oven and bake for 8-10 minutes, or until salmon is cooked through.

6. In a small saucepan, melt butter over medium heat.

7. Add minced garlic and sauté for 1 minute.

8. Stir in lemon juice, dill, and white wine (or broth). Cook for 2-3 minutes until slightly thickened.

9. Serve salmon fillets with the lemon dill sauce drizzled over the top.

2. Shrimp and Vegetable Stir-Fry

Prep Time: 15 minutes
Cook Time: 10 minutes
Total Time: 25 minutes
Servings: 4

Ingredients:

- 1 lb shrimp, peeled and deveined
- 2 tablespoons coconut oil or avocado oil
- 1 red bell pepper, sliced
- 1 cup broccoli florets
- 1 cup sliced mushrooms
- 2 cloves garlic, minced

The Balanced Balanced Body compass

- 1 teaspoon grated fresh ginger
- 2 tablespoons coconut aminos or tamari sauce
- 1 tablespoon rice vinegar
- Salt and pepper to taste
- Chopped green onions for garnish

Nutritional Information (per serving):

Calories: 240,Total Fat: 10g,Saturated Fat: 4g
Cholesterol: 185mg,Sodium: 830mg
Total Carbohydrates: 12g,Dietary Fiber: 3g
Protein: 25g

Instructions:

1. In a large skillet or wok, heat coconut oil or avocado oil over high heat.
2. Add sliced bell pepper, broccoli florets, and sliced mushrooms. Stir-fry for 2-3 minutes.
3. Add minced garlic and grated ginger. Stir-fry for 1 minute until fragrant.
4. Add shrimp and continue stir-frying for 3-4 minutes until shrimp are pink and opaque.
5. Stir in coconut aminos (or tamari sauce) and rice vinegar. Season with salt and pepper to taste.
6. Garnish with chopped green onions and serve hot over cauliflower rice or zucchini noodles.

The Balanced Balanced Body compass

3. Cod with Tomato and Olive Tapenade

Prep Time: 15 minutes
Cook Time: 15 minutes
Total Time: 30 minutes
Servings: 4

- Ingredients:
- 4 (6 oz) cod fillets
- Salt and pepper to taste
- 2 tablespoons olive oil
- 1 cup cherry tomatoes, halved
- 1/2 cup pitted Kalamata olives, chopped
- 2 cloves garlic, minced
- 2 tablespoons capers
- 1 tablespoon lemon juice
- 2 tablespoons chopped fresh parsley

Nutritional Information (per serving):

Calories: 280,Total Fat: 13g,Saturated Fat: 2g
Cholesterol: 60mg,Sodium: 530mg
Total Carbohydrates: 6g,Dietary Fiber: 1g
Protein: 33g

Instructions:

1. Preheat oven to 400°F (200°C).
2. Season cod fillets with salt and pepper.
3. Heat olive oil in an oven-safe skillet over medium-high heat.
4. Sear cod fillets for 2 minutes per side until lightly browned.
5. Transfer skillet to the preheated oven and bake for 8-10 minutes, or until cod is cooked through.
6. In a small bowl, combine cherry tomatoes, chopped olives, minced garlic, capers, lemon juice, and chopped parsley.
7. Top the baked cod fillets with the tomato and olive tapenade.
8. Serve hot, with roasted vegetables or a side salad if desired.

4. Grilled Tuna Steaks with Mango Salsa

Prep Time: 20 minutes
Cook Time: 10 minutes
Total Time: 30 minutes
Servings: 4

Ingredients:

The Balanced Balanced Body compass

- 4 (6 oz) tuna steaks
- 2 tablespoons olive oil
- Salt and pepper to taste

For the Mango Salsa:

- 1 ripe mango, diced
- 1/2 red onion, finely chopped
- 1 jalapeño, seeded and minced
- 2 tablespoons lime juice
- 2 tablespoons chopped fresh cilantro
- Salt to taste

Nutritional Information (per serving):

Calories: 320,Total Fat: 12g,Saturated Fat: 2g
Cholesterol: 60mg,Sodium: 180mg
Total Carbohydrates: 17g,Dietary Fiber: 2g
Protein: 36g

Instructions:

1. Preheat grill or grill pan to medium-high heat.
2. Brush tuna steaks with olive oil and season with salt and pepper.

The Balanced Balanced Body compass

3. Grill tuna steaks for 3-4 minutes per side for rare, or until desired doneness.

4. While tuna is grilling, prepare the mango salsa by combining diced mango, chopped red onion, minced jalapeño, lime juice, chopped cilantro, and salt in a bowl.

5. Serve grilled tuna steaks hot, topped with the mango salsa.

6. Optionally, serve with a side of cauliflower rice or roasted vegetables.

Potato and sweet potato sides

1. Roasted Sweet Potato Wedges

Prep Time: 10 minutes
Cook Time: 30 minutes
Total Time: 40 minutes
Servings: 4

Ingredients:

The Balanced Balanced Body compass

- 4 medium sweet potatoes, cut into wedges
- 2 tablespoons olive oil
- 1 teaspoon paprika
- 1 teaspoon garlic powder
- 1/2 teaspoon salt
- 1/4 teaspoon black pepper

Nutritional Information (per serving):

Calories: 190, Total Fat: 7g, Saturated Fat: 1g
Cholesterol: 0mg, Sodium: 300mg
Total Carbohydrates: 31g, Dietary Fiber: 5g
Protein: 2g

Instructions:

1. Preheat oven to 400°F (200°C).
2. In a large bowl, toss the sweet potato wedges with olive oil, paprika, garlic powder, salt, and black pepper until evenly coated.
3. Arrange the seasoned wedges in a single layer on a baking sheet lined with parchment paper or a silicone mat.
4. Roast in the preheated oven for 25-30 minutes, flipping halfway through, until tender and crispy on the outside.

The Balanced Balanced Body compass

5. Serve hot, garnished with chopped fresh parsley or chives if desired.

2. Garlic Mashed Potatoes

Prep Time: 10 minutes
Cook Time: 20 minutes
Total Time: 30 minutes
Servings: 4

Ingredients:

- 2 lbs russet potatoes, peeled and quartered
- 4 tablespoons butter or ghee
- 1/2 cup warm unsweetened almond milk or broth
- 4 cloves garlic, minced
- Salt and pepper to taste

Nutritional Information (per serving):

Calories: 260,Total Fat: 13g,Saturated Fat: 8g
Cholesterol: 30mg,Sodium: 120mg
Total Carbohydrates: 34g,Dietary Fiber: 3g
Protein: 4g

Instructions:

1. Place the quartered potatoes in a large pot and cover with water. Bring to a boil over high heat.
2. Reduce heat to medium-low and simmer for 15-20 minutes, or until potatoes are tender when pierced with a fork.
3. Drain the potatoes and return them to the pot.
4. Add butter (or ghee), warm almond milk (or broth), and minced garlic to the pot.
5. Mash the potatoes with a potato masher or an electric hand mixer until smooth and creamy.
6. Season with salt and pepper to taste.
7. Serve hot, garnished with chopped fresh parsley or chives if desired.

3. Twice-Baked Loaded Sweet Potatoes

Prep Time: 15 minutes
Cook Time: 1 hour 15 minutes
Total Time: 1 hour 30 minutes
Servings: 4

Ingredients:
- 4 medium sweet potatoes
- 1/4 cup butter or ghee, softened

- 1/4 cup full-fat coconut milk or dairy-free milk
- 1/4 cup crumbled cooked bacon (optional)
- 2 green onions, sliced
- Salt and pepper to taste

Nutritional Information (per serving):

Calories: 340,Total Fat: 18g,Saturated Fat: 11g
Cholesterol: 30mg, Sodium: 260mg
Total Carbohydrates: 41g,Dietary Fiber: 6g
Protein: 5g

Instructions:

1. Preheat oven to 400°F (200°C).
2. Scrub the sweet potatoes and prick them several times with a fork.
3. Place the sweet potatoes on a baking sheet and bake for 45-60 minutes, or until tender when pierced with a fork.
4. Remove from the oven and let cool slightly. Reduce oven temperature to 350°F (175°C).
5. Slice the sweet potatoes in half lengthwise and scoop out the flesh into a large bowl, leaving a thin layer of flesh attached to the skins.

6. Add butter (or ghee), coconut milk (or dairy-free milk), crumbled bacon (if using), and sliced green onions to the bowl with the sweet potato flesh.

7. Mash the mixture until well combined and season with salt and pepper to taste.

8. Spoon the mashed sweet potato mixture back into the potato skins.

9. Place the stuffed potato halves on a baking sheet and bake for an additional 15-20 minutes, or until heated through and lightly browned on top.

10. Serve hot, garnished with additional green onions or chopped chives if desired.

4. Crispy Smashed Potatoes

Prep Time: 10 minutes
Cook Time: 30 minutes
Total Time: 40 minutes
Servings: 4

Ingredients:

- 1 lb baby potatoes or small red potatoes
- 2 tablespoons olive oil
- 1 teaspoon garlic powder
- 1/2 teaspoon paprika

The Balanced Balanced Body compass

- 1/2 teaspoon salt
- 1/4 teaspoon black pepper

Nutritional Information (per serving):

Calories: 170,Total Fat: 7g,Saturated Fat: 1g
Cholesterol: 0mg,Sodium: 380mg
Total Carbohydrates: 26g,Dietary Fiber: 3g
Protein: 3g

Instructions:

1. Preheat oven to 450°F (230°C).
2. Place the baby potatoes or small red potatoes in a large pot and cover with water. Bring to a boil over high heat.
3. Reduce heat to medium-low and simmer for 10-12 minutes, or until potatoes are tender when pierced with a fork.
4. Drain the potatoes and let cool slightly.
5. Place the cooked potatoes on a baking sheet lined with parchment paper or a silicone mat. Using a potato masher or the bottom of a glass, gently smash each potato until it's about 1/2-inch thick.

6. Drizzle the smashed potatoes with olive oil and sprinkle with garlic powder, paprika, salt, and black pepper.

7. Roast in the preheated oven for 20-25 minutes, or until crispy on the outside and golden brown.

8. Serve hot, garnished with chopped fresh parsley or chives if desired.

Sauces, condiments, and dressings

1. Chimichurri Sauce

Prep Time: 10 minutes
Cook Time: 0 minutes
Total Time: 10 minutes
Servings: 8 (2 tablespoons per serving)

Ingredients:

- 1 cup fresh parsley, packed
- 1/2 cup olive oil
- 1/4 cup red wine vinegar

- 4 cloves garlic, minced
- 2 tablespoons fresh oregano, chopped
- 1 teaspoon red pepper flakes
- 1/2 teaspoon salt
- 1 1/4 teaspoon black pepper

Nutritional Information (per serving):

Calories: 120,Total Fat: 14g,Saturated Fat: 2g
Cholesterol: 0mg,Sodium: 110mg
Total Carbohydrates: 1g,Dietary Fiber: 0g
Protein: 0g

Instructions:

1. In a food processor or blender, combine all the ingredients and pulse until well combined but still slightly chunky.
2. Adjust seasoning with salt and pepper to taste.
3. Transfer to an airtight container and refrigerate until ready to use.

2. Dairy-Free Ranch Dressing

Prep Time: 10 minutes
Cook Time: 0 minutes

The Balanced Balanced Body compass

Total Time: 10 minutes
Servings: 8 (2 tablespoons per serving)

Ingredients:

- 1 cup cashew butter
- 1/2 cup unsweetened almond milk
- 2 tablespoons lemon juice
- 2 tablespoons apple cider vinegar
- 1 clove garlic, minced
- 1 teaspoon dried dill
- 1 teaspoon dried chives
- 1/2 teaspoon onion powder
- 1/2 teaspoon salt
- 1/4 teaspoon black pepper

Nutritional Information (per serving):

Calories: 150,Total Fat: 12g,Saturated Fat: 2g
Cholesterol: 0mg,Sodium: 210mg
Total Carbohydrates: 6g,Dietary Fiber: 1g
Protein: 4g

Instructions:

1. In a blender or food processor, combine all the ingredients and blend until smooth and creamy.
2. Adjust seasoning with salt and pepper to taste.
3. Transfer to an airtight container and refrigerate until ready to use.

3. Balsamic Vinaigrette

Prep Time: 5 minutes
Cook Time: 0 minutes
Total Time: 5 minutes
Servings: 8 (2 tablespoons per serving)

Ingredients:

- 1/2 cup olive oil
- 1/4 cup balsamic vinegar
- 1 tablespoon Dijon mustard
- 1 clove garlic, minced
- 1 teaspoon honey (optional)
- 1/2 teaspoon salt
- 1/4 teaspoon black pepper

Nutritional Information (per serving):

Calories: 120,Total Fat: 14g,Saturated Fat: 2g

The Balanced Balanced Body compass

Cholesterol: 0mg,Sodium: 190mg
Total Carbohydrates: 2g,Dietary Fiber: 0g
Protein: 0g

Instructions:

1. In a small bowl or jar with a tight-fitting lid, combine all the ingredients.
2. Whisk or shake vigorously until well combined and emulsified.
3. Adjust seasoning with salt and pepper to taste.
4. Refrigerate until ready to use.

4. Guacamole

Prep Time: 10 minutes
Cook Time: 0 minutes
Total Time: 10 minutes
Servings: 8 (1/4 cup per serving)

Ingredients:

- 3 ripe avocados, pitted and mashed
- 1/4 cup diced red onion
- 2 tablespoons fresh lime juice
- 1 jalapeño, seeded and minced

The Balanced Balanced Body compass

- 1/4 cup chopped fresh cilantro
- 1/2 teaspoon salt
- 1/4 teaspoon black pepper

Nutritional Information (per serving):

Calories: 120, Total Fat: 11g,Saturated Fat: 2g
Cholesterol: 0mg,Sodium: 150mg
Total Carbohydrates: 6g, Dietary Fiber: 4g
Protein: 1g

Instructions:

1. In a medium bowl, mash the avocados with a fork or potato masher until slightly chunky.
2. Add the diced red onion, lime juice, minced jalapeño, chopped cilantro, salt, and black pepper.
3. Gently mix until well combined.
4. Adjust seasoning with salt and pepper to taste.
5. Serve immediately or refrigerate until ready to use.

dairy-free dressings and sauces

1. Tahini Dressing

The Balanced Balanced Body compass

Prep Time: 5 minutes
Cook Time: 0 minutes
Total Time: 5 minutes
Servings: 8 (2 tablespoons per serving)

Ingredients:

- 1/2 cup tahini
- 1/4 cup lemon juice
- 1/4 cup water
- 2 cloves garlic, minced
- 1 teaspoon maple syrup (optional)
- 1/2 teaspoon salt
- 1/4 teaspoon black pepper

Nutritional Information (per serving):

Calories: 100,Total Fat: 9g,Saturated Fat: 1g
Cholesterol: 0mg,Sodium: 160mg
Total Carbohydrates: 4g,Dietary Fiber: 1g
Protein: 3g

Instructions:

1. In a small bowl, whisk together all the ingredients until smooth and well combined.
2. Adjust seasoning with salt and pepper to taste.
3. If the dressing is too thick, add a tablespoon or two of water to reach your desired consistency.
4. Refrigerate until ready to use.

2. Cashew Cream Sauce

Prep Time: 5 minutes
Cook Time: 0 minutes
Total Time: 5 minutes
Servings: 4 (1/4 cup per serving)

Ingredients:

- 1 cup raw cashews, soaked in water for at least 4 hours or overnight
- 1/2 cup unsweetened almond milk
- 2 tablespoons lemon juice
- 1 clove garlic, minced
- 1/2 teaspoon salt
- 1/4 teaspoon black pepper

Nutritional Information (per serving):

Calories: 210,Total Fat: 17g,Saturated Fat: 3g,

The Balanced Balanced Body compass

Cholesterol: 0mg,Sodium: 300mg
Total Carbohydrates: 10g,Dietary Fiber: 1g
Protein: 6g

Instructions:

1. Drain and rinse the soaked cashews.
2. In a high-speed blender or food processor, combine the cashews, almond milk, lemon juice, garlic, salt, and black pepper.
3. Blend until smooth and creamy, scraping down the sides as needed.
4. Adjust seasoning with salt and pepper to taste.
5. Use immediately or refrigerate until ready to use.

3. Avocado Cilantro Dressing

Prep Time: 10 minutes
Cook Time: 0 minutes
Total Time: 10 minutes
Servings: 8 (2 tablespoons per serving)

Ingredients:

- 1 ripe avocado, pitted and peeled
- 1/4 cup olive oil

The Balanced Balanced Body compass

- 1/4 cup water
- 2 tablespoons fresh lime juice
- 1/2 cup fresh cilantro leaves
- 1 clove garlic, minced
- 1/2 teaspoon salt
- 1/4 teaspoon black pepper

Nutritional Information (per serving):

Calories: 110,Total Fat: 11g,Saturated Fat: 1.5g
Cholesterol: 0mg,Sodium: 140mg
Total Carbohydrates: 3g,Dietary Fiber: 2g
Protein: 1g

Instructions:

1. In a blender or food processor, combine all the ingredients and blend until smooth and creamy.
2. Adjust seasoning with salt and pepper to taste.
3. If the dressing is too thick, add a tablespoon or two of water to reach your desired consistency.
4. Refrigerate until ready to use.

4. Teriyaki Sauce

Prep Time: 5 minutes

The Balanced Balanced Body compass

Cook Time: 5 minutes
Total Time: 10 minutes
Servings: 8 (2 tablespoons per serving)

Ingredients:

- 1/2 cup coconut aminos or tamari sauce
- 1/4 cup rice vinegar
- 2 tablespoons maple syrup
- 2 cloves garlic, minced
- 1 teaspoon grated fresh ginger
- 1 teaspoon sesame oil
- 1/4 teaspoon red pepper flakes (optional)
- 2 tablespoons water
- 1 tablespoon arrowroot powder or cornstarch

Nutritional Information (per serving):

Calories: 30, Total Fat: 1g, Saturated Fat: 0g, Cholesterol: 0mg, Sodium: 540mg, Total Carbohydrates: 6g,
Dietary Fiber: 0g, Protein: 1g

Instructions:

The Balanced Balanced Body compass

1. In a small saucepan, whisk together the coconut aminos (or tamari), rice vinegar, maple syrup, minced garlic, grated ginger, sesame oil, and red pepper flakes (if using).

2. In a small bowl, whisk together the water and arrowroot powder (or cornstarch) to make a slurry.

3. Bring the sauce mixture to a simmer over medium heat. Whisk in the slurry and continue cooking for 1-2 minutes, or until the sauce thickens slightly.

4. Remove from heat and let cool slightly.

5. Transfer to an airtight container and refrigerate until ready to use.

Nut-free condiments

1. Pesto (Nut-Free)

Prep Time: 10 minutes
Cook Time: 0 minutes
Total Time: 10 minutes
Servings: 8 (2 tablespoons per serving)

Ingredients:

- 2 cups fresh basil leaves
- 1/2 cup olive oil
- 1/4 cup nutritional yeast
- 2 cloves garlic, minced
- 2 tablespoons lemon juice
- 1/2 teaspoon salt
- 1/4 teaspoon black pepper

Nutritional Information (per serving):

Calories: 120,Total Fat: 14g,Saturated Fat: 2g
Cholesterol: 0mg,Sodium: 150mg
Total Carbohydrates: 1g,Dietary Fiber: 0g
Protein: 1g

Instructions:

1. In a food processor or blender, combine the basil leaves, olive oil, nutritional yeast, minced garlic, lemon juice, salt, and black pepper.
2. Pulse until the mixture is well combined and reaches the desired consistency, scraping down the sides as needed.
3. Adjust seasoning with salt and pepper to taste.
4. Transfer to an airtight container and refrigerate until ready to use.

The Balanced Balanced Body compass

2. Tomato Jam

Prep Time: 10 minutes
Cook Time: 45 minutes
Total Time: 55 minutes
Servings: 16 (2 tablespoons per serving)

Ingredients:

- 2 lbs ripe tomatoes, diced
- 1/2 cup sugar or maple syrup
- 2 tablespoons apple cider vinegar
- 1 teaspoon ground ginger
- 1/2 teaspoon ground cinnamon
- 1/4 teaspoon ground cloves
- 1/4 teaspoon salt

Nutritional Information (per serving):

Calories: 40,Total Fat: 0g,Saturated Fat: 0g
Cholesterol: 0mg,Sodium: 60mg
Total Carbohydrates: 10g,Dietary Fiber: 1g
Protein: 0g

Instructions:

The Balanced Balanced Body compass

1. In a large saucepan, combine the diced tomatoes, sugar (or maple syrup), apple cider vinegar, ground ginger, cinnamon, cloves, and salt.

2. Bring the mixture to a simmer over medium heat, stirring occasionally.

3. Reduce heat to low and continue simmering for 35-45 minutes, stirring frequently, until the mixture has thickened and reached a jam-like consistency.

4. Remove from heat and let cool slightly.

5. Transfer the tomato jam to an airtight container and refrigerate until ready to use.

3. Coconut Bacon Bits

Prep Time: 5 minutes
Cook Time: 15 minutes
Total Time: 20 minutes
Servings: 8 (2 tablespoons per serving)

Ingredients:

- 1 cup unsweetened coconut flakes
- 2 tablespoons coconut aminos or tamari sauce
- 1 tablespoon maple syrup
- 1 teaspoon liquid smoke (optional)

The Balanced Balanced Body compass

- 1/2 teaspoon smoked paprika
- 1/4 teaspoon salt

Nutritional Information (per serving):

Calories: 90,Total Fat: 7g,Saturated Fat: 6g
Cholesterol: 0mg, Sodium: 160mg
Total Carbohydrates: 6g,Dietary Fiber: 2g
Protein: 1g

Instructions:

1. Preheat oven to 325°F (165°C). Line a baking sheet with parchment paper.
2. In a small bowl, mix together the coconut flakes, coconut aminos (or tamari sauce), maple syrup, liquid smoke (if using), smoked paprika, and salt until well combined.
3. Spread the coconut mixture in an even layer on the prepared baking sheet.
4. Bake for 12-15 minutes, stirring occasionally, until the coconut flakes are crispy and lightly browned.
5. Remove from oven and let cool completely.
6. Store the coconut bacon bits in an airtight container at room temperature for up to 1 week.

The Balanced Balanced Body compass

4. Garlic Herb Sauce

Prep Time: 10 minutes
Cook Time: 0 minutes
Total Time: 10 minutes
Servings: 8 (2 tablespoons per serving)

Ingredients:

- 1 cup fresh parsley leaves
- 1/2 cup olive oil
- 1/4 cup water
- 2 cloves garlic, minced
- 2 tablespoons lemon juice
- 1 teaspoon dried oregano
- 1/2 teaspoon salt
- 1/4 teaspoon black pepper

Nutritional Information (per serving):

Calories: 100,Total Fat: 11g,Saturated Fat: 1.5g
Cholesterol: 0mg,Sodium: 150mg
,Total Carbohydrates: 1g,Dietary Fiber: 0g,Protein:
0g

The Balanced Balanced Body compass

Instructions:

1. In a blender or food processor, combine the parsley leaves, olive oil, water, minced garlic, lemon juice, dried oregano, salt, and black pepper.
2. Blend until smooth and well combined, scraping down the sides as needed.
3. Adjust seasoning with salt and pepper to taste.
4. Transfer to an airtight container and refrigerate until ready to use.

Dips and spreads

1. Hummus

Prep Time: 10 minutes
Cook Time: 0 minutes
Total Time: 10 minutes
Servings: 8 (1/4 cup per serving)

Ingredients:

- 1 (15 oz) can chickpeas, drained and rinsed
- 1/4 cup tahini

The Balanced Balanced Body compass

- 1/4 cup lemon juice
- 2 cloves garlic, minced
- 2 tablespoons olive oil
- 1 teaspoon ground cumin
- 1/2 teaspoon salt
- 1/4 cup water (or more, as needed)

Nutritional Information (per serving):

Calories: 150,Total Fat: 9g,Saturated Fat: 1g
Cholesterol: 0mg,Sodium: 230mg
Total Carbohydrates: 14g,Dietary Fiber: 4g
Protein: 5g

Instructions:

1. In a food processor or blender, combine the chickpeas, tahini, lemon juice, minced garlic, olive oil, cumin, and salt.
2. Pulse until the mixture is well combined, adding water as needed to reach the desired consistency.
3. Taste and adjust seasoning with salt and lemon juice if needed.
4. Transfer to a serving bowl and refrigerate until ready to serve.

The Balanced Balanced Body compass

2. Baba Ghanoush

Prep Time: 15 minutes
Cook Time: 30 minutes
Total Time: 45 minutes
Servings: 8 (1/4 cup per serving)

Ingredients:

- 1 large eggplant
- 2 tablespoons tahini
- 2 tablespoons lemon juice
- 2 cloves garlic, minced
- 2 tablespoons olive oil
- 1/4 cup fresh parsley, chopped
- 1 teaspoon ground cumin
- 1/2 teaspoon salt
- 1/4 teaspoon black pepper

Nutritional Information (per serving):

Calories: 80, Total Fat: 6g,Saturated Fat: 1g
Cholesterol: 0mg, Sodium: 150mg
Total Carbohydrates: 7g,Dietary Fiber: 3g
Protein: 1g

The Balanced Balanced Body compass

Instructions:

1. Preheat oven to 400°F (200°C).
2. Prick the eggplant a few times with a fork and place it on a baking sheet.
3. Roast the eggplant for 30-35 minutes, or until it's very soft and the skin is charred.
4. Let the roasted eggplant cool slightly, then scoop out the flesh and transfer it to a food processor or blender.
5. Add the tahini, lemon juice, minced garlic, olive oil, chopped parsley, cumin, salt, and black pepper.
6. Pulse until the mixture is well combined and reaches the desired consistency, scraping down the sides as needed.
7. Taste and adjust seasoning with salt and lemon juice if needed.
8. Transfer to a serving bowl and refrigerate until ready to serve.

3. White Bean Dip

Prep Time: 10 minutes
Cook Time: 0 minutes
Total Time: 10 minutes
Servings: 8 (1/4 cup per serving)

The Balanced Balanced Body compass

Ingredients:

- 1 (15 oz) can white beans, drained and rinsed
- 1/4 cup olive oil
- 2 tablespoons lemon juice
- 2 cloves garlic, minced
- 1 teaspoon dried rosemary
- 1/2 teaspoon salt
- 1/4 teaspoon black pepper

Nutritional Information (per serving):

Calories: 120,Total Fat: 8g,Saturated Fat: 1g
Cholesterol: 0mg,Sodium: 200mg
Total Carbohydrates: 10g,Dietary Fiber: 3g
Protein: 3g

Instructions:

1. In a food processor or blender, combine the white beans, olive oil, lemon juice, minced garlic, dried rosemary, salt, and black pepper.
2. Pulse until the mixture is well combined and reaches the desired consistency, scraping down the sides as needed.

3. Taste and adjust seasoning with salt and lemon juice if needed.

4. Transfer to a serving bowl and refrigerate until ready to serve.

4. Roasted Red Pepper Spread

Prep Time: 10 minutes
Cook Time: 0 minutes
Total Time: 10 minutes
Servings: 8 (2 tablespoons per serving)

Ingredients:

- 1 (12 oz) jar roasted red peppers, drained
- 1/4 cup olive oil
- 2 tablespoons lemon juice
- 2 cloves garlic, minced
- 1/4 cup fresh basil leaves
- 1/2 teaspoon salt
- 1/4 teaspoon black pepper

Nutritional Information (per serving):

Calories: 90,Total Fat: 9g,Saturated Fat: 1g
Cholesterol: 0mg,Sodium: 190mg

The Balanced Balanced Body compass

Total Carbohydrates: 3g,Dietary Fiber: 1g
Protein: 1g

Instructions:

1. In a food processor or blender, combine the roasted red peppers, olive oil, lemon juice, minced garlic, fresh basil leaves, salt, and black pepper.
2. Pulse until the mixture is well combined and reaches the desired consistency, scraping down the sides as needed.
3. Taste and adjust seasoning with salt and lemon juice if needed.
4. Transfer to a serving bowl and refrigerate until ready to serve.

Fruit-Based treats, beverages, and teas

1. Chia Seed Pudding with Mixed Berries

Prep Time: 10 minutes (plus 4-6 hours chilling time)

The Balanced Balanced Body compass

Cook Time: 0 minutes
Total Time: 4-6 hours
Servings: 4

Ingredients:

- 1/4 cup chia seeds
- 1 cup unsweetened almond milk or coconut milk
- 1 tablespoon maple syrup or honey (optional)
- 1 teaspoon vanilla extract
- 1 cup mixed berries (e.g., strawberries, blueberries, raspberries)

Nutritional Information (per serving):

Calories: 120,Total Fat: 5g,Saturated Fat: 0.5g
Cholesterol: 0mg,Sodium: 45mg
Total Carbohydrates: 15g,Dietary Fiber: 8g
 Protein: 4g

Instructions:

1. In a medium bowl, combine the chia seeds, almond milk (or coconut milk), maple syrup (or honey, if using), and vanilla extract. Whisk well to combine.

2. Cover the bowl and refrigerate for 4-6 hours or overnight, until the chia seeds have absorbed the liquid and formed a pudding-like consistency.

3. Divide the chia seed pudding into individual bowls or glasses.

4. Top with fresh mixed berries and serve chilled.

2. Strawberry Chia Fresca

Prep Time: 10 minutes
Cook Time: 0 minutes
Total Time: 10 minutes
Servings: 4

Ingredients:

- 1 cup fresh strawberries, hulled and sliced
- 1/4 cup chia seeds
- 4 cups water
- 2 tablespoons fresh lime juice
- 2 tablespoons honey or maple syrup (optional)

Nutritional Information (per serving):

Calories: 80,Total Fat: 3g,Saturated Fat: 0g

Cholesterol: 0mg, Sodium: 10mg
Total Carbohydrates: 13g, Dietary Fiber: 6g
Protein: 2g

Instructions:

1. In a large pitcher or jar, combine the sliced strawberries, chia seeds, water, lime juice, and honey (or maple syrup, if using). Stir well to combine.
2. Refrigerate for at least 30 minutes, or until the chia seeds have absorbed the liquid and formed a gel-like consistency.
3. Stir the mixture before serving and adjust sweetness if desired.
4. Pour into glasses and serve chilled.

3. Hibiscus Iced Tea

Prep Time: 5 minutes
Cook Time: 10 minutes
Total Time: 15 minutes
Servings: 4

Ingredients:

- 4 cups water

The Balanced Balanced Body compass

- 1/4 cup dried hibiscus flowers
- 2 tablespoons honey or maple syrup (optional)
- Fresh mint leaves for garnish (optional)

Nutritional Information (per serving):

Calories: 0, Total Fat: 0g, Saturated Fat: 0g
Cholesterol: 0mg, Sodium: 0mg
 Total Carbohydrates: 0g,Dietary Fiber: 0g
Protein: 0g

Instructions:

1. In a small saucepan, bring the water to a boil over high heat.
2. Remove the saucepan from heat and add the dried hibiscus flowers. Cover and let steep for 10 minutes.
3. Strain the tea through a fine-mesh sieve to remove the hibiscus flowers.
4. Stir in honey or maple syrup if desired.
5. Let the tea cool to room temperature, then refrigerate until chilled.
6. Serve over ice, garnished with fresh mint leaves if desired.

The Balanced Balanced Body compass

4. Watermelon Lime Smoothie

Prep Time: 5 minutes
Cook Time: 0 minutes
Total Time: 5 minutes
Servings: 2

Ingredients:

- 2 cups cubed seedless watermelon
- 1/2 cup unsweetened almond milk or coconut milk
- 1/2 cup plain Greek yogurt or dairy-free yogurt
- 2 tablespoons fresh lime juice
- 1 tablespoon honey or maple syrup (optional)

Nutritional Information (per serving):

Calories: 120,Total Fat: 2g
Saturated Fat: 0g,Cholesterol: 0mg (if using dairy-free yogurt),Sodium: 45mg
Total Carbohydrates: 23g, Dietary Fiber: 1g,
Protein: 4g

Instructions:

The Balanced Balanced Body compass

1. In a blender, combine the cubed watermelon, almond milk (or coconut milk), Greek yogurt (or dairy-free yogurt), lime juice, and honey (or maple syrup, if using).
2. Blend on high speed until smooth and creamy.
3. Pour the smoothie into glasses and serve chilled.

Anti-Inflammatory Chia Seed Pudding recipe:

Preparation Time: 5 minutes
Cooking Time: None (just need to chill)
Total Time: 5 minutes + 2-3 hours chilling
Serves: 2

Ingredients:

- 1/4 cup chia seeds
- 1 cup unsweetened almond milk or coconut milk
- 1 tsp ground cinnamon
- 1/2 tsp vanilla extract

The Balanced Balanced Body compass

- 1-2 tbsp maple syrup or honey (optional, to taste)
- 1/2 cup fresh or frozen berries (such as blueberries, raspberries, strawberries)

Instructions:

1. In a bowl or jar, combine the chia seeds, almond/coconut milk, cinnamon, vanilla, and sweetener if using.
2. Whisk well to combine and break up any clumps of chia seeds.
3. Cover and refrigerate for 2-3 hours or overnight, until thickened to a pudding-like consistency.
4. Once thickened, give it a stir and portion into serving bowls or glasses.
5. Top with fresh or frozen berries.

Nutritional Value (Per Serving):

Calories: 210,Total Fat: 10g,Saturated Fat: 1g
Cholesterol: 0mg,Sodium: 115mg
Total Carbohydrates: 24g,Dietary Fiber: 11g
Total Sugars: 8g,Protein: 6g

1. Coconut Mango Chia Pudding

Prep Time: 5 minutes
Chilling Time: 2-3 hours
Servings: 2

Ingredients:

- 1/4 cup chia seeds
- 1 cup coconut milk
- 1/2 cup diced mango
- 1 tsp vanilla extract
- 1 tbsp honey (optional)
- Toasted coconut flakes for topping

Instructions:

Combine all ingredients except mango. Chill for 2-3 hours to thicken. Top with diced mango and coconut flakes.

2. Chocolate Avocado Chia Pudding

Prep Time: 10 minutes
Chilling Time: 2-3 hours
Servings: 2

The Balanced Balanced Body compass

Ingredients:

- 1/4 cup chia seeds
- 1 ripe avocado, mashed
- 1 cup unsweetened almond milk
- 2 tbsp cocoa powder
- 1 tsp vanilla
- 2 tbsp maple syrup

Instructions:

Blend all ingredients except chia seeds until smooth. Stir in chia seeds. Chill for 2-3 hours to thicken.

3. Pumpkin Pie Chia Pudding

Prep Time: 5 minutes
Chilling Time: 2-3 hours
Servings: 2

Ingredients:

- 1/4 cup chia seeds
- 1 cup coconut milk
- 1/2 cup pumpkin puree

The Balanced Balanced Body compass

- 1 tsp pumpkin pie spice
- 1 tbsp maple syrup
- Pecans for topping

Instructions:

Whisk all ingredients together. Chill 2-3 hours to thicken. Top with pecans.

4. Matcha Green Tea Chia Pudding

Prep Time: 5 minutes
Chilling Time: 2-3 hours
Servings: 2

Ingredients:

- 1/4 cup chia seeds
- 1 cup unsweetened almond milk
- 1 tsp matcha green tea powder
- 1/2 tsp vanilla extract
- Diced kiwi for topping

Instructions:

Whisk all ingredients except kiwi until well combined. Chill 2-3 hours to thicken. Top with diced kiwi.

hydrating herbal tea blends:

1. Lemon Ginger Herbal Tea

Prep Time: 5 minutes
Cook Time: 5-7 minutes
Total Time: 10-12 minutes
Servings: 1

Ingredients:

- 1 cup water
- 1 inch fresh ginger, sliced
- 1/2 lemon, juiced
- 1 tsp honey (optional)

Instructions:

1. In a small saucepan, bring water to a boil.
2. Add sliced ginger and allow to simmer for 5-7 minutes.

3. Remove from heat and stir in lemon juice and honey if using.

4. Strain into a mug and enjoy hot or iced.

Nutrition per serving:

Calories: 15,Fiber: 0.2g,Protein: 0.1g

2. Hibiscus Berry Herbal Tea

Prep Time: 2 minutes
Steep Time: 5-7 minutes
Servings: 1

Ingredients:

- 1 hibiscus tea bag
- 1/2 cup hot water
- 1/2 cup cold water or ice
- 1 tbsp fresh or frozen berries

Instructions:

1. Steep hibiscus tea bag in 1/2 cup hot water for 5-7 minutes.

2. Remove tea bag and add 1/2 cup cold water or ice.

3. Stir in berries.

Nutrition per serving:

Calories: 2 ,Fiber: 1g

3. Peppermint Lavender Iced Tea

Prep Time: 2 minutes
Steep Time: 5-7 minutes
Servings: 1

Ingredients:

- 1 peppermint tea bag
- 1 tsp dried lavender flowers
- 1 cup hot water
- Ice

Instructions:

1. Steep peppermint tea bag and lavender in 1 cup hot water for 5-7 minutes.
2. Remove tea bag and lavender.
3. Pour over ice and enjoy.

Nutrition per serving:

Calories: 0, Fiber: 0g

No added sugars or calories makes these herbal teas a perfect hydrating beverage on the anti-inflammatory diet. They provide antioxidants and can aid digestion.

4. Turmeric Ginger Lemongrass Tea

Prep Time: 5 minutes
Steep Time: 5-7 minutes
Servings: 1

Ingredients:

- 1 inch fresh turmeric, grated or sliced
- 1 inch fresh ginger, grated or sliced
- 2 lemongrass stalks, bruised
- 1 cup hot water
- Honey to taste (optional)

Instructions:

The Balanced Balanced Body compass

1. Combine turmeric, ginger, and lemongrass in a mug or teapot.
2. Pour in hot water and allow to steep for 5-7 minutes.
3. Strain into a cup and add honey if desired.

Nutrition per serving:

Calories: 6,Fiber: 0.5g

5. Rose Hibiscus Mint Tea

Prep Time: 2 minutes
Steep Time: 5-7 minutes
Servings: 1

Ingredients:

- 1 hibiscus tea bag
- 1 tsp dried rose petals
- 3-4 fresh mint leaves
- 1 cup hot water

Instructions:
1. Place hibiscus tea bag, rose petals and mint in a mug or teapot.

2. Pour hot water over and steep for 5-7 minutes.
3. Remove tea bag and stir gently before drinking.

Nutrition per serving:
Calories: 0,Fiber: 1g

Chapter 2

28-Day

Meal Plan

The Balanced Balanced Body compass

weekly meal plans and shopping lists for the 28-day meal plan:

Week 1 Meal Plan:

Breakfast: Banana Coconut Smoothie, Sweet Potato Hash with Sautéed Greens, Avocado Boats with Baked Eggs

Lunch: Zucchini Noodle Salad with Lemon Vinaigrette, Curried Chicken Salad Lettuce Wraps, Carrot Ginger Soup

Dinner: Baked Salmon with Roasted Brussels Sprouts, Beef and Vegetable Stir-Fry over Cauliflower Rice, Stuffed Portobello Mushrooms

Snacks: Fresh Fruit, Coconut Butter, Cucumber, Guacamole, Sugar-free Beef Jerky

Week 1 Shopping List:

The Balanced Balanced Body compass

Produce: Bananas, sweet potatoes, greens, avocados, zucchini, lemons, carrots, ginger, brussels sprouts, cauliflower, portobello mushrooms, fruit, cucumbers
Protein: Eggs, salmon, chicken, beef
Other: Coconut milk, coconut butter, olive oil, vinegar, curry powder, beef jerky

Week 2 Meal Plan:

Breakfast: Pumpkin Spice Smoothie, Mini Frittata Muffins, Plantain Pancakes with Berry Compote
Lunch: Thai Salad with Ginger Dressing, Loaded Sweet Potato with Chicken, Tuna Avocado Lettuce Wraps
Dinner: Garlic Lemon Shrimp with Zucchini Noodles, Korean Beef Bowl with Cauliflower Rice, Moroccan Chicken with Roasted Vegetables
Snacks: Apples, cinnamon, coconut butter, plantains, hard boiled eggs

Week 2 Shopping List:

Produce: Pumpkin puree, eggs, plantains, berries, greens, ginger, sweet potatoes, avocados, zucchini, cauliflower, mixed vegetables, apples
Protein: Chicken, tuna, shrimp, beef
Other: Coconut milk, Thai curry paste, lemon, coconut butter, cinnamon

Week 3 Meal Plan:

Breakfast: Breakfast Hash with Sweet Potatoes and Bacon, Coconut Flour Pancakes with Maple Cranberries, Smoked Salmon Avocado Boats

Lunch: Zucchini Noodle Chicken Alfredo, Lettuce Cups with Kalua Pulled Pork, Tomato Soup with Crispy Prosciutto

Dinner: Meatballs with Marinara over Spaghetti Squash, Shepherd's Pie with Cauliflower Mash, Chicken Fajitas with Jicama Tortillas

Snacks: Eggs, grapes, cashews, coconut yogurt, berries

Week 3 Shopping List:

Produce: Sweet potatoes, bacon, cranberries, avocados, smoked salmon, zucchini, lettuce, tomatoes, prosciutto, spaghetti squash, cauliflower, mixed peppers, onions, jicama, grapes, berries

Protein: Eggs, pulled pork, ground beef/turkey, chicken

Other: Coconut flour, maple syrup, marinara sauce, coconut yogurt, cashews

Week 4 Meal Plan:

The Balanced Balanced Body compass

Breakfast: Mexican Breakfast Casserole, Indian Spiced Chia Pudding, Japanese Sweet Potato Pancakes
Lunch: Greek Salad with Lemon Dill Dressing, Peruvian Chicken Soup, Veggie Spring Rolls with Ginger Lime Sauce
Dinner: Caribbean Jerk Chicken with Mango Salsa, Italian Bolognese over Zucchini Noodles, Middle Eastern Lamb Meatballs with Cauliflower Tabbouleh
Snacks: Melon, mint, chickpeas, pepitas (pumpkin seeds)

Week 4 Shopping List:

Produce: Sweet potatoes, greens, tomatoes, onions, mangoes, zucchini, cauliflower, parsley, mint, melon, limes, ginger, mixed veggies for rolls
Protein: Eggs, chicken, ground lamb, canned chickpeas
Other: Chia seeds, Greek olives/feta (omit for AIP), lemon, dill, jerk seasoning, Italian spices, pepitas.

Sample meal combinations using the recipes from the 28-day meal plan:

Week 1:

Breakfast: Sweet Potato Hash with Sautéed Greens
Lunch: Curried Chicken Salad Lettuce Wraps with a side of Carrot Ginger Soup
Dinner: Baked Salmon with Roasted Brussels Sprouts and Zucchini Noodle Salad with Lemon Vinaigrette
Snack: Fresh Fruit with Coconut Butter

Week 2:

Breakfast: Plantain Pancakes with Berry Compote
Lunch: Thai Salad with Ginger Dressing and Tuna Avocado Lettuce Wraps
Dinner: Korean Beef Bowl with Cauliflower Rice and Garlic Lemon Shrimp with Zucchini Noodles
Snack: Apple Slices with Cinnamon Coconut Butter

Week 3:

Breakfast: Coconut Flour Pancakes with Maple Cranberries and Smoked Salmon Avocado Boats
Lunch: Zucchini Noodle Chicken Alfredo with a side salad
Dinner: Shepherd's Pie with Cauliflower Mash and roasted vegetables
Snack: Deviled Eggs and Grapes with Cashews

Week 4:

Breakfast: Mexican Breakfast Casserole
Lunch: Peruvian Chicken Soup and Veggie Spring Rolls with Ginger Lime Sauce
Dinner: Caribbean Jerk Chicken with Mango Salsa, Middle Eastern Lamb Meatballs and Cauliflower Tabbouleh
Snack: Melon Skewers with Mint and Roasted Chickpeas

Tips for batch cooking and prep on the AIP diet:

Batch Cook Proteins:
• Grill, bake or instant pot a large batch of chicken breasts, turkey burgers or ground meat to use throughout the week in salads, lettuce wraps, stir-fries etc.
• Bake a few salmon filets or other fish at once to have protein ready to go.
• Cook a large pork or beef roast and slice up to use for multiple meals.

Prep Vegetables:
• Wash and cut up a variety of raw veggies like carrots, celery, cucumber, broccoli, cauliflower etc. for easy snacking or cooking later.
• Roast a few pans of vegetables like brussels sprouts, sweet potatoes and beets to have ready for meals.
• Make a batch of zucchini noodles or cauliflower rice to use as bases for dishes.

Make Sauces/Dressings:

The Balanced Balanced Body compass

• Blend up a double batch of pesto, ranch, vinaigrettes or other compliant sauces/dressings to have on hand.
• Make a big pot of marinara, curry sauce or soup to portion out.

Bake Ahead:
• Make muffins, breads, pancakes or waffles in batches to freeze for quick AIP-friendly breakfasts.
• Bake a few frittata or breakfast casserole dishes to have slices ready to reheat.

Snacks:
• Dehydrate plantains or bake a batch of plantain chips.
• Make a big batch of trail mix with coconut chips, nuts/seeds and dried fruit.
• Hard boil a dozen eggs to have ready as snacks or salad toppers.

Having basics prepped makes throwing together AIP meals easier during the week. Cooking once and batch prepping sets you up for success!

Reference

Pahwa, R., & Jialal, I. (2019). Chronic inflammation. In: StatPearls [Internet]. Treasure Island (FL): StatPearls Publishing.

Minihane, A. M., Vinoy, S., Russell, W. R., Baka, A., Roche, H. M., Tuohy, K. M., ... & Calder, P. C. (2015). Low-grade inflammation, diet composition and health: current research evidence and its translation. British Journal of Nutrition, 114(7), 999-1012.

Konijeti, G. G., Kim, N., Lewis, J. D., Groven, S., Chandrasekaran, A., Grandhe, S., ... & Tanoue, M. T. (2017). Efficacy of the autoimmune protocol diet for inflammatory bowel disease. Inflammatory bowel diseases, 23(11), 2054-2060.

Ballantyne, S. (2013). The paleo approach: reverse autoimmune disease and heal your body. Victory Belt Publishing.

Printed in Great Britain
by Amazon